DR. R.M.P. KAWONGA

19: 02: 03.

atlas of
Clinical
Hematology

Douglas C. Tkachuk, MD

Chief of Hematology and Coagulation,
Pathology and Laboratory Service
Puget Sound VA Medical Center
Assistant Professor of Pathology
University of Washington School of Medicine
Seattle, Washington

J. V. Hirschmann, MD

Assistant Chief, Medical Service
Puget Sound VA Medical Center
Professor of Medicine
University of Washington School of Medicine
Seattle, Washington

James R. McArthur, MD

Emeritus Professor of Medicine, Hematology
Former Director, American Society of Hematology Slide Bank
University of Washington School of Medicine
Seattle, Washington

W.B. SAUNDERS COMPANY
A Harcourt Health Sciences Company
Philadelphia   London   New York   Sydney   St. Louis   Toronto

W.B. Saunders Company
A Division of Harcourt Brace & Company

The Curtis Center
Independence Square West
Philadelphia, Pennsylvania 19106

Library of Congress Cataloging in Publication Data

Tkachuk, Douglas C.
  Atlas of clinical hematology / Douglas C. Tkachuk,
J.V. Hirschmann, James R. McArthur.—1st ed.
      p.   cm.
    ISBN 0-7216-7002-4
    1. Blood—Diseases Atlases. 2. Hematology Atlases.
I. Hirschmann, Jan V. II. McArthur, James R., 1930–   .
III. Title.
    [DNLM: 1. Hematology—methods Atlases. 2. Hematologic
Diseases—diagnosis Atlases. WH 17 T626a 2002]
RB145.T56   2002
616.1′5—dc21
DNLM/DLC
for Library of Congress   99-37692
                                                                CIP

ATLAS OF CLINICAL HEMATOLOGY   0–7216–7002–4

Printed in China

Last digit is the print number: 9   8   7   6   5   4   3   2   1

PREFACE

The purpose of this text-atlas is to provide excellent images and written descriptions of peripheral blood smears, bone marrow aspirates, and bone marrow biopsies from normal adults and those with common hematologic abnormalities. An introductory section provides information on the examination of these hematologic preparations, and, to help readers understand the various manifestations of the diseases, a lengthy section of text discusses individual disorders, with brief summaries of the important clinical and pathophysiologic features. The tables list the most common causes of the conditions mentioned, rather than being exhaustive compilations.

The atlas intentionally includes some repetition because readers will likely refer to discrete sections rather than read the material consecutively. The book concentrates on common disorders and the routine stains used in daily hematologic practice. Accordingly, it does not include specimens prepared with immunohistochemical staining procedures. Also excluded is treatment information, which is a rapidly changing area for many of the disorders discussed. The proposed audience consists of anyone interested in blood diseases, including medical students, physicians in training, and laboratory technicians, as well as hematologists.

The images in the atlas came from two major sources. One is the large number of photographs, taken specifically for this atlas, of specimens from patients at the Puget Sound Veterans Administration Medical Center in Seattle. The other primary source is the third edition of the Slide Bank of the American Society of Hematology. Housed at the University of Washington School of Medicine in Seattle, the slides in this repository consist of reviewed photographs submitted by hematologists from around the world. The following figures are used with permission from that source: slides 7, 8, 12, 16, 18, 21–23, 26, 34, 40, 41, 60, 65, 66, 73, 74, 78, 87, 94, 95, 98, 102, 104, 106, 125–127, 133–140, 147, 148, 154, 155, 160, 166–168, 171–173, 176, 177, 181, and 182. We appreciate the generosity of those who originally submitted material to this collection. We also would like to thank E. Dale Everett, M.D., for slide 165, which originally appeared in *Current Opinion in Infectious Diseases* (1996; 23:314), and David Spach, M.D., and Thomas Fritsche, M.D., for slide 174, published in the *New England Journal of Medicine* (1993; 329:944). Both are reproduced here with the permission of those journals. Photographs from all these sources were transformed into digital images and slight alterations were made to eliminate artifacts, improve and standardize the color, magnify the cells, if necessary, and delete extraneous material when appropriate. The presence of Dr. McArthur as a coauthor of this atlas does not imply endorsement by the American Society of Hematology.

We are very grateful for the generous assistance of Eden Palmer and Karna McKinney at the Puget Sound Veterans Administration Medical Center, who helped with the photomicroscopy and image preparation, respectively, and Joseph Wilmhoff at the University of Washington School of Medicine, who assisted us with the digital imaging.

Slide Preparation and Staining

A smear is prepared by placing a drop of blood on a slide and spreading it across the glass surface with the edge of another slide. An alternative is to put a drop of blood on a coverslip, place another coverslip over the first, allow the blood to spread, and then slide the coverslips apart by pulling them in opposite directions. Instead of coverslips, slides can be used. In a third method, done by machine, the slide with a drop of blood on it is spun; the centrifugal force spreads the blood across the glass surface.

Staining the slide, now usually performed by automated hematology analyzers, employs a mixture of dyes first used by Romanowsky, a Russian protozoologist, who in 1890 combined eosin with moldy, old methylene blue to stain the nucleus of a malarial parasite purple and its cytoplasm blue. Subsequent modifications include the May-Grünwald-Giemsa stain, widely used in Europe and the United Kingdom, and the Wright stain, the most common preparation in the United States. Both contain eosin and methylene azures, which are derivatives of methylene blue. The alkaline methylene azures give a blue to bluish-purple color to acidic components of the cell, including nucleic acids (RNA and DNA), nucleoproteins, and the granules of basophils, whose acid ingredient is heparin. The acidic eosin reacts with the basic elements of the cell, such as hemoglobin and the granules of eosinophils (which contain a strongly alkaline spermine derivative), coloring them red or orange.

Slide Examination

A properly stained blood smear has a pinkish hue. When it is excessively blue, the cause may be too thick a film, a problem with the dyes, or too long a staining time. When one smear is considerably darker than others made with the same batch, high levels of plasma proteins, as in multiple myeloma, must be considered.

On microscopic examination, one should first view the slide at low power (using the 10 or 20× objective) and then at higher power (40 or 50× objective) before switching to oil immersion. At these lower magnifications the examiner can survey the film rapidly to detect abnormalities in cell number, type, or aggregation and to find the best area in which to examine the cells in more detail. For erythrocytes, the optimal region is where they are in a monolayer with cells close to each other but not overlapping. White cells, however, are sometimes most numerous, and best examined, at the edges of the film.

CONTENTS

THE PERIPHERAL SMEAR

Evaluation of Red Cells

In evaluating red cells the examiner looks for abnormalities in size and shape, hemoglobin content, inclusions, aggregation, and immature forms. The normal red cell is about 8 μm in diameter, slightly less than the nucleus of a small lymphocyte, which is approximately 8.5 μm. When the erythrocyte's size is normal, it is *normocytic;* when larger, *macrocytic;* and when smaller, *microcytic.* The automated cell counters measure size as mean cell volume (MCV); microcytosis corresponds to an MCV < 80 fl, macrocytosis to an MCV > 100 fl. A substantial variation in size is called *anisocytosis* and registers on the automated counters as an increased red cell distribution width (RDW).

The biconcave erythrocyte is thinner in the middle, creating a central pallor on blood smears that is ordinarily less than ⅓ of the cell's diameter. Such a cell, possessing the normal amount of hemoglobin, is called *normochromic.* When the central pallor is greater than normal, indicating decreased hemoglobin content, the erythrocyte is *hypochromic.* Severe hypochromia corresponds to a decreased mean cell hemoglobin concentration (MCHC) as measured by the automated analyzers. When central pallor is absent from cells that are separated from contiguous ones, the usual reason is a decrease in cell membrane surface, making the cell denser, less concave in the center, and more spherical, hence a *spherocyte.* Some macrocytic cells are thicker than normal and also lack central pallor.

The examiner should look for abnormalities in red cell shape (a significant increase in the number of abnormally shaped cells is called *poikilocytosis*) and scrutinize the interior of the erythrocytes to detect inclusions and the presence of nuclei or a bluish-purple color, indicating immature cells. Finally, the examiner looks for abnormalities in red cell aggregation—*agglutination,* or the clumping of red cells into a rosette configuration, or *rouleaux,* erythrocytes aligned in a row like a stack of coins.

NORMAL RED CELLS

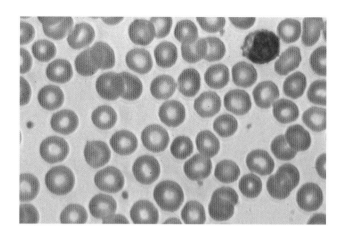

Slide 1. Normal Red Cells

The red cells are fairly uniform in size and shape. Central pallor is present but constitutes less than ⅓ of the erythrocyte's diameter (about 8 μm), which is slightly less than that of the nucleus of the small lymphocyte (about 8.5 μm) (also see slide 34). The red cells are thus normal in hemoglobin content (*normochromic*) and size (*normocytic*).

ABNORMALITIES IN RED CELL SIZE AND HEMOGLOBIN CONTENT

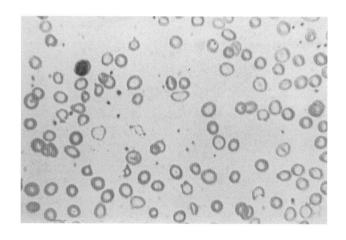

Slide 2. Microcytic, Hypochromic Red Cells

Many of the erythrocytes are smaller than the nucleus of the small lymphocyte and have markedly increased central pallor, exceeding ⅓ the diameter of the red cell. The erythrocytes, therefore, are microcytic (<7.0 μm in diameter) and hypochromic. These features, which usually coexist, indicate abnormal hemoglobin synthesis. The major causes are iron deficiency, thalassemias, hemoglobinopathies, some sideroblastic anemias, and the anemia of chronic disease, in which microcytosis occurs in about 20% of cases. In addition to microcytosis and hypochromia, the erythrocytes in this slide exhibit variation in size (anisocytosis) and shape (poikilocytosis). This patient had iron deficiency anemia, which accounts for the increased number of platelets.

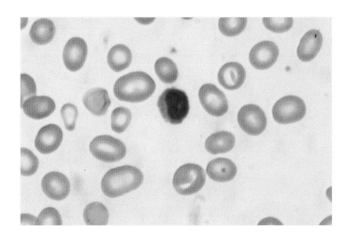

Slide 3. Macrocytic Red Cells

Most of the red cells are larger than the nucleus of the small lymphocyte. The erythrocytes are therefore macrocytic (>8.5 μm in diameter). The major causes of macrocytic red cells are alcoholism, liver disease, vitamin B_{12} or folate deficiency, myelodysplastic syndromes, hypothyroidism, drugs that impair folate or DNA synthesis, and blood loss or hemolysis. The increased erythrocyte size in blood loss or hemolysis arises from the presence of large, immature forms released early from the bone marrow in response to intense erythropoietin stimulus. Some of these young erythrocytes differ from mature red cells on Romanowsky stains only by their size; others are identifiable by their bluish–gray color, called polychromatophilia or polychromasia (see slide 19).

The presence of oval macrocytes (macro–ovalocytes) in this slide strongly suggests myelodysplasia or a deficiency in folate or vitamin B_{12}; in other disorders causing macrocytosis, the large erythrocytes are uniformly round. Note the variation in red cell size and shape. This patient had vitamin B_{12} deficiency.

Slide 4. Spherocyte

Spherocytes form because an inherited or acquired defect in the erythrocyte membrane decreases the surface area to volume ratio. Because a sphere's diameter is less than that of a disk-shaped object containing the same volume, the spherocytes are typically smaller than mature red cells. Hereditary spherocytosis is most often an autosomal dominant disease, but about 25% of cases arise from de novo mutations. Transfused erythrocytes are often spherocytic, and transfusion is the most common cause of spherocytes in clinical practice. The other major cause of numerous spherocytes is warm-antibody hemolytic anemia, in which the spleen removes small portions of the red cell membrane from cells coated with IgG antibodies. The erythrocyte then emerges from the spleen as a smaller cell with a decreased surface area to volume ratio (microcytic and lacking central pallor). Since the normal amount of hemoglobin is concentrated into a smaller cell, the erythrocyte appears hyperchromic. This change is reflected in an increased mean cell hemoglobin content (MCHC) on automated counters, and many cases of autoimmune hemolytic anemia are initially suspected from the elevated MCHC. Unusual causes of spherocytes include severe burns, in which very small cells (microspherocytes) are typically present, or toxin damage from bacterial sepsis caused by *Clostridium perfringens*. The examiner should look for spherocytes in areas of the blood smear where the cells do not overlap, because normal erythrocytes may resemble spherocytes at the edges of slides, although in that location they are usually broad, pale, and somewhat square.

This slide, from a patient with warm-antibody autoimmune hemolytic anemia, shows several spherocytes, with an especially prominent one in the middle. They are small cells lacking central pallor. Many normocytic cells with central pallor are also present, as is typical in this disorder.

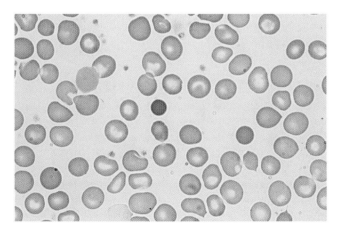

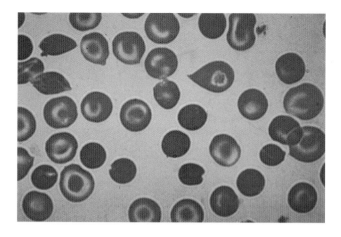

pallor. This configuration occurs from an increase in the red cell membrane compared to the hemoglobin content (an increased surface area to volume ratio), the opposite of what happens with spherocytes. When the erythrocytes dry on the slide, the excess membrane pools in the middle of the cells. The cause of target cells may be diminished hemoglobin content from iron deficiency, hemoglobinopathies, and thalassemias; in these disorders the cells are typically microcytic. Target cells can also occur from obstructive jaundice or primary hepatocellular diseases such as hepatitis, in which the cell membrane enlarges by abnormally incorporating lipids, creating target cells that are usually normocytic or macrocytic. Normocytic target cells may also be present in hyposplenism and some hemoglobinopathies. This slide, from a patient with combined β-thalassemia and hemoglobin C disease, contains prominent target cells, numerous spherocytes in the center of the slide, and two bite cells (see slide 11) in the lower center.

Slide 5. Target Cells

In target cells the erythrocyte's center contains a circle of hemoglobin pigment surrounded by a ring of

ABNORMALITIES IN RED CELL SHAPE

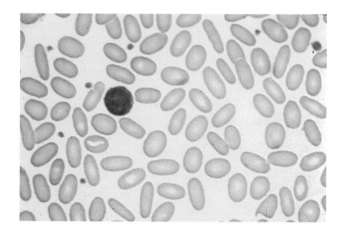

Slide 6. Elliptocyte

Red cells may be elliptical in various anemias, especially macrocytic ones. In a group of hereditary, usually autosomal dominant, disorders, elliptocytes constitute at least 25% of the erythrocytes, hemolysis is usually mild, and anemia is present in only about 5–20% of cases. This slide, from a patient with hereditary elliptocytosis, discloses red cells that are dark and lack central pallor. In iron deficiency anemia elongated erythrocytes ("pencil cells") may form, but, unlike elliptocytes, they are thin and pale.

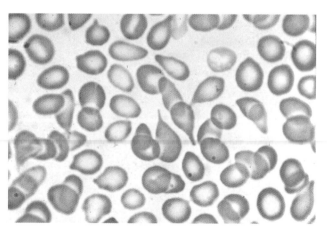

Slide 7. Teardrop Cell (Dacryocyte)

These pear-shaped cells, seen most prominently in thalassemias and diseases involving bone marrow infiltration by fibrosis or malignancy, apparently form from distortion of the erythrocytes as they travel through the vasculature of an abnormal bone marrow or spleen. Good examples, present in the center of this slide, illustrate that the pointed ends may be sharp or blunt.

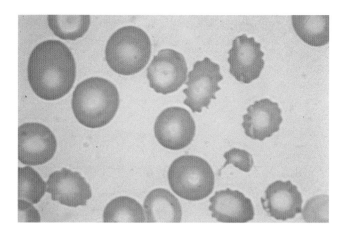

Slide 8. Burr Cells (Echinocytes)

Burr cells usually have 10–30 blunt and fairly symmetrical projections. They are prominent in renal failure from any cause and may also occur with liver diseases, especially when uremia coexists. Burr cells can also develop as a storage artifact if blood is kept in a tube for several hours before preparation of the smear. The mechanism of echinocyte formation is unknown; perhaps an increase in fatty acids alters the cell membrane.

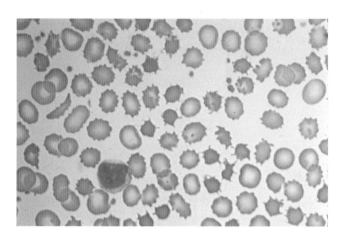

Slide 9. Spur Cells (Acanthocytes)

Because of changes in membrane lipid content, these red cells have several irregularly distributed, sharp projections of unequal length. Most of the affected erythrocytes are also small and lack central pallor. Acanthocytes are prominent in spur-cell anemia, where liver disease, usually alcoholic cirrhosis, causes an increase in the cholesterol:phospholipid ratio in the red cell membrane, leading to hemolysis, which is usually severe. Acanthocytosis also occurs in abetalipoproteinemia, a rare autosomal recessive disorder of lipid metabolism characterized by fat malabsorption, retinitis pigmentosa, anemia, and ataxia. Spur cells are a diagnostic feature of neuroacanthocytosis, a disease that may be hereditary or nonfamilial; its major features are personality change, progressive intellectual deterioration, and a movement disorder, most commonly chorea.

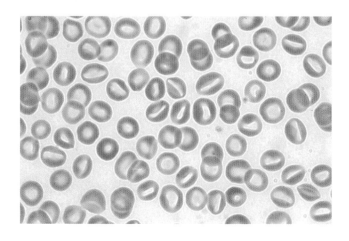

Slide 10. Stomatocytes

On wet preparations the stomatocyte, rather than being biconcave like normal erythrocytes, is concave on only one side, resembling a cup or bowl. When examined on dry smears, it has a central slit or stoma (mouth). A few stomatocytes may be present in normal people, occasionally constituting >5% of the erythrocytes. Conditions associated with this abnormality of the red cell membrane include alcoholism, liver disease, malignancies, various cardiovascular and pulmonary disorders, treatment with certain drugs, and an autosomal dominant disorder in which stomatocytes constitute 10–50% of the circulating erythrocytes, hemolysis is mild, and anemia is slight or absent. This slide is from a patient with alcoholic liver disease.

Slide 11. Bite Cell (Degmacyte)

Bite cells have a semicircular defect in their edge that resembles a bite mark. These defects occur when certain drugs cause oxidative destruction of hemoglobin, often in patients with a deficiency of the enzyme glucose-6-phosphate dehydrogenase (G6PD). Heinz bodies, which are erythrocyte inclusions of denatured hemoglobin, result, but they are not visible on Romanowsky stains. They are detectable when dyes such as methyl or cresyl violet, new methylene blue, or brilliant cresyl blue are mixed with unfixed cells before microscopic examination (see slide 104). Because the erythrocytes are still alive when the dye is added, the preparations are called "supravital" stains. The bite cells apparently occur when the spleen removes the Heinz bodies from the erythrocytes. Other features of severe oxidative injury visible on Romanowsky stains include "ghost cells," in which the erythrocyte is nearly devoid of pigment, and hemi-ghost cells, in which hemoglobin is present in only one half of the cell. A bite cell lies in the center of this slide from a patient who developed hemolytic anemia after receiving phenazopyridine (Pyridium) for a urinary tract infection. Basophilic stippling is also present (see slide 15).

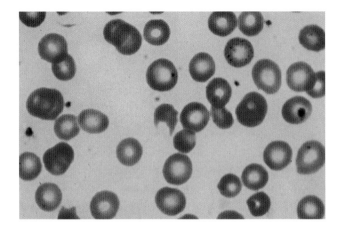

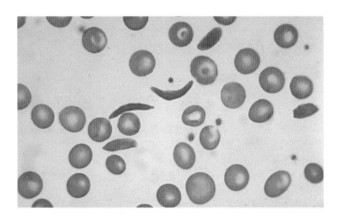

Slide 12. Sickle Cells

Crescent-shaped sickle cells develop in people homozygous for the hemoglobin S (HbS) gene (see slide 97) and in those heterozygous for HbS and either a thalassemia or another abnormal hemoglobin such as HbC (see slide 99). Patients with sickle cell trait—heterozygous for HbS and HbA—do not have sickle cells. In addition to the sickle cells, this slide demonstrates target cells and polychromatophilia (bluish-purple color) in the large erythrocyte at the bottom of the slide (see slide 19).

Slide 13. Schistocytes

Physical trauma to erythrocytes within the bloodstream can create fragments called schistocytes, which include such strange forms as helmet cells, triangles, crescents, and microspherocytes. These malformed cells may occur as a complication of prosthetic cardiac valves, especially the aortic valve, in which regurgitation is usually present; the red cells are probably sheared by turbulent blood flow. Schistocytes also develop in microangiopathic hemolytic anemia, a term for a group of disorders in which injury to red cells occurs as they traverse strands of intravascular fibrin or travel across an irregular, damaged endothelial surface. Causes of microangiopathic hemolytic anemia include the hemolytic-uremic syndrome, thrombotic thrombocytopenic purpura, disseminated carcinoma (especially gastric), chemotherapy (especially with mitomycin C), malignant hypertension, and disseminated intravascular coagulation of any cause. This slide, from a patient with disseminated intravascular coagulation, demonstrates numerous fragments and irregularly shaped erythrocytes. Platelets are absent.

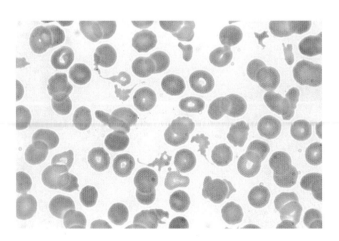

RED CELL INCLUSIONS

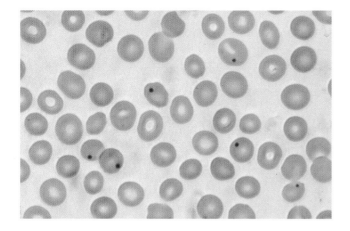

Slide 14. Howell-Jolly Bodies

Howell-Jolly bodies are round, purple inclusions in erythrocytes that represent DNA fragments that were once part of the nucleus of immature red cells. Usually only one inclusion is present per cell, and, because the spleen normally removes them, Howell-Jolly bodies are not typically visible on peripheral blood smears. They are universally present in patients with absent or hypofunctioning spleens, although the number of cells with these inclusions varies from sparse to abundant. They occasionally occur with increased red cell production, such as in macrocytic or hemolytic anemias. Single Howell-Jolly bodies are present in several erythrocytes throughout this slide from a patient who had undergone a splenectomy.

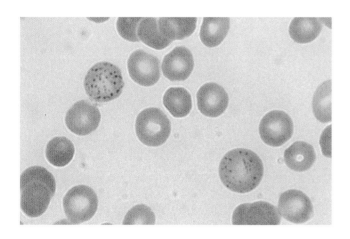

Slide 15. Basophilic Stippling

Basophilic stippling is the presence of numerous small, purplish inclusions within erythrocytes that represent aggregates of ribosomal RNA. It occurs with defective hemoglobin synthesis, as in lead poisoning, thalassemias, hemoglobinopathies, and macrocytic anemias. It is commonly present in polychromatophilic cells (see slide 19). Its presence argues against iron deficiency. Basophilic stippling is apparent in two erythrocytes in this slide from a patient with lead poisoning.

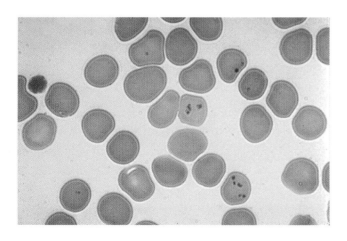

Slide 16. Pappenheimer Bodies

Pappenheimer bodies are dark blue granules, usually irregular in size and shape, that tend to occur in small clusters, predominantly in the cell periphery. These iron-containing inclusions are visible on Romanowsky stains because they are partially composed of ribosomal RNA. Their iron constitution is demonstrable on Perls' or Prussian blue stains. Erythrocytes with Pappenheimer bodies are called siderocytes, and they are present following splenectomy and in hemolytic anemias, myelodysplastic syndromes, lead poisoning, and sideroblastic anemias. Their presence is a strong argument against iron deficiency.

ABNORMALITIES IN RED CELL AGGREGATION

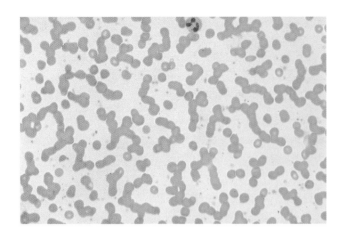

Slide 17. Rouleaux

Rouleaux occur when red cells adhere in a pattern resembling a stack of coins. Erythrocytes, being nega-tively charged, ordinarily repel one another. With abnormal or excessive amounts of positively charged proteins, the red cells stick together and form rouleaux. Important causes include high levels of monoclonal immunoglobulins, as in multiple myeloma or Waldenström's macroglobulinemia; pregnancy (because of increased fibrinogen); and inflammatory disorders, in which polyclonal immunoglobulins, α_2-macroglobulins, and fibrinogen are elevated or abnormal. Rouleaux may also occur with erythrocytosis. Examination for rouleaux formation, best done at low magnification, must be in a thin portion of the slide where the cells do not ordinarily overlap. Even in healthy people, rouleaux are common in thick portions of a blood smear where erythrocytes become superimposed. This slide, photographed at low power and from a patient with multiple myeloma, reveals the typical appearance of rouleaux—red cells arrayed in rows of adherent cells.

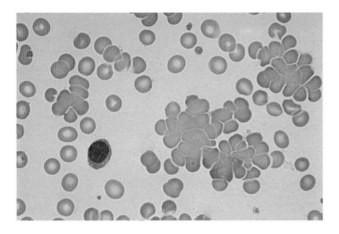

Slide 18. Red Cell Agglutination

When coated with antibodies, erythrocytes can form irregular clumps. A small amount of such agglutination may occur in warm-antibody (IgG) hemolytic anemia. More extensive clumping typically develops with high levels of IgM, which are present in Waldenström's macroglobulinemia or in cold-agglutinin hemolytic anemia from such causes as infectious mononucleosis and *Mycoplasma pneumoniae* infection. This slide, from a patient with chronic idiopathic cold-agglutinin disease, demonstrates large aggregates of clumped red cells.

IMMATURE RED CELLS

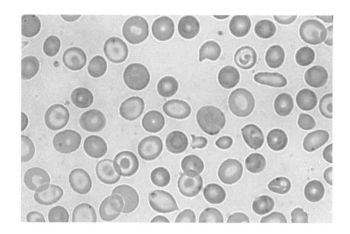

Slide 19. Polychromatophilia (Polychromasia)

Most immature, non-nucleated red cells are indistinguishable by size or color from mature erythrocytes on Romanowsky stains. When dyes such as new methylene blue or brilliant cresyl blue are mixed with unfixed cells when the cells are still alive, the preparations are called supravital stains. With these preparations, the ribosomes of immature erythrocytes become visible in a reticular pattern. Such cells are called reticulocytes (see slide 91). Some very early

reticulocytes, which are larger than mature erythrocytes, are detectable on Romanowsky preparations because the substantial residual RNA in the cells stains a bluish-gray or purple. This phenomenon is called polychromatophilia or polychromasia (more than one color), because the cells' hue derives from the combination of blue from the RNA and red from the hemoglobin. A few polychromatophilic cells are present on normal smears. When diseases such as metastatic malignancy disrupt the normal bone marrow architecture or when high levels of erythropoietin circulate as a response to the presence of an anemia, increased numbers of these erythrocytes, often called "shift cells," may appear in the peripheral circulation. The absence of polychromatophilic cells in a normocytic, normochromic anemia suggests a hypoproliferative disorder in which either erythropoietin is diminished (e.g., chronic renal failure) or the bone marrow is unresponsive to it (e.g., pure red cell aplasia). Polychromatophilic cells are also common with asplenia. They have no central pallor, and basophilic stippling is often present. In this slide two polychromatophilic cells appear as purplish, large cells lacking central pallor. Numerous target cells are present, as are some microcytes and an elliptocyte.

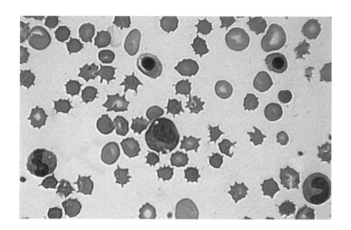

Slide 20. Nucleated Red Cells

Except in newborns, nucleated red cells are abnormal in the peripheral blood. They may appear in response to marked stimulation of the bone marrow by erythropoietin in patients with severe anemias or from disruption of the bone marrow by infiltrating disorders such as myelofibrosis or metastatic malignancy. The nucleated erythrocyte has a dark, dense nucleus in the center of a bluish (polychromatophilic) or red (orthochromatic) cell. Two nucleated red cells are visible in this slide from a patient who had alcoholic liver disease, as evidenced by the numerous acanthocytes (see slides 9 and 103), and a myeloproliferative syndrome. There are three large granulated cells—a neutrophil, a myelocyte (in the center of the slide), and a band (see slides 21, 22, and 65).

Evaluation of White Cells

An important part of examining white cells is to assess the frequency of the various kinds of granulocytic, lymphoid, and monocytic cells. Other elements to scrutinize include the appearance of the nucleus, the nature of any granules or inclusions in the cytoplasm, and the presence of immature forms.

NORMAL NEUTROPHILS

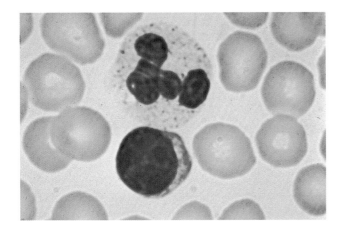

Slide 21. Mature Neutrophil

The mature neutrophil or polymorphonuclear leukocyte ("poly") is about 12–15 μm in diameter. The nucleus normally contains condensed, dark-staining material arranged in two to five lobes joined together by thick threads of chromatin. Fine violet-pink granules appear throughout the pink cytoplasm. In this slide a mature neutrophil with four lobes abuts a normal lymphocyte.

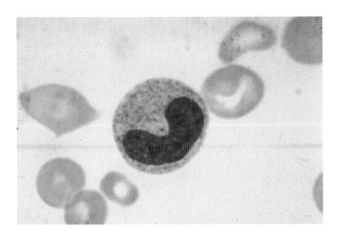

Slide 22. Band (Juvenile or Stab Forms)

Normally, bands constitute <5–10% of the white cells. They differ from mature neutrophils primarily in having a curved or coiled nucleus of consistent width, which, although sometimes indented, does not segment into lobes. Distinguishing between mature neutrophils and bands is often difficult because the lobes of neutrophils may overlap and obscure their connecting filaments. Consequently, interobserver variability in enumerating bands is common. An increase in the number of bands and other immature neutrophils is called a "shift to the left" and can occur in many situations, including infections, noninfectious inflammatory diseases, and uncomplicated pregnancy.

ABNORMAL NUCLEI IN NEUTROPHILS

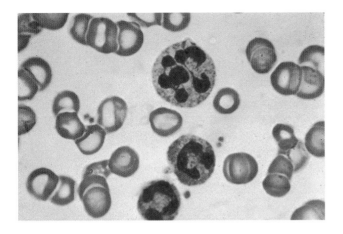

Slide 23. Hypersegmented Neutrophil

The normal number of lobes in neutrophils is two to five, the average being about three. Hypersegmentation exists when >5% of neutrophils have five lobes or when any have six or more lobes. Such hypersegmentation is common in folate and vitamin B_{12} deficiency and can be present in myelodysplastic and myeloproliferative disorders. When enlarged, neutrophils with increased segmentation are called *macropolycytes*. The largest neutrophil in this slide, from a patient with pernicious anemia (vitamin B_{12} deficiency), has seven lobes.

Slide 24. Pelger-Huët Anomaly

Reduced neutrophil segmentation can occur as an autosomal dominant disorder, the Pelger-Huët anomaly, in which 70–90% of the neutrophils have hypolobulated, rounded nuclei with condensed chroma-

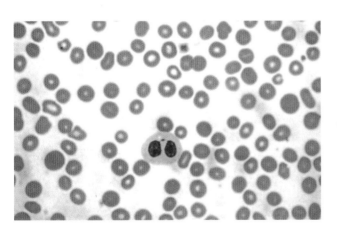

tin. A thin strand of chromatin may connect the lobes, creating a pince-nez (spectacle) shape, or a larger bridge can give the nucleus a peanut appearance. A few neutrophils have only one nucleus, but they differ from immature forms (myelocytes) (see slide 65) by the presence of small nuclei, condensed chromatin, and mature cytoplasm. This hereditary hypolobulation has no clinical significance, and no other hematologic abnormalities coexist.

An acquired (pseudo-Pelger-Huët) anomaly, common in myelodysplastic and myeloproliferative syndromes (see later discussions of these conditions), is distinguishable from the inherited disorder in that the percentage of affected neutrophils is smaller, the cytoplasm is often hypogranular, neutropenia is frequent, and Döhle bodies (see slide 28) may be present. The neutrophil in this slide, from a patient with myelodysplasia, is bilobed, with a pince-nez appearance.

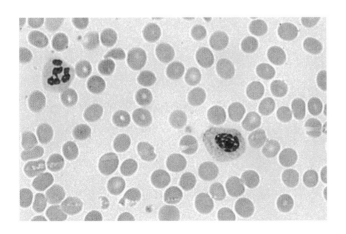

Slide 25. Hypolobulated Neutrophil

As indicated in the previous slide, hypolobulation of neutrophils occurs in the Pelger-Huët anomaly or in myelodysplasia, where hypersegmented neutrophils may also appear. Other conditions in which it develops include acute or chronic granulocytic leukemia, idiopathic myelofibrosis, therapy with certain drugs, and a few other disorders. In this slide, from a patient with myelodysplasia, a neutrophil with a single nucleus is on the right of the slide; on the left is a neutrophil containing five lobes. Near the hypolobulated neutrophil is a scratch artifact coursing through five erythrocytes.

ABNORMALITIES OF NEUTROPHIL GRANULES

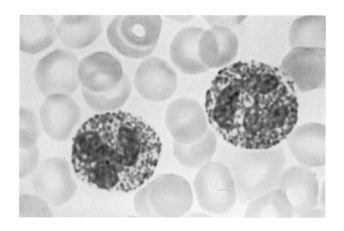

Slide 26. Toxic Granulation

Toxic granulation indicates the presence of increased numbers of granules that are larger and more basophilic than normal. It may occur from treatment with colony-stimulating factors, during pregnancy, or as an accompaniment of several disorders, including severe infections (especially bacterial), burns, malignancies, drug reactions, aplastic anemia, and the hypereosinophilic syndrome. Both neutrophils in this slide demonstrate toxic granulation, which almost obscures the nucleus.

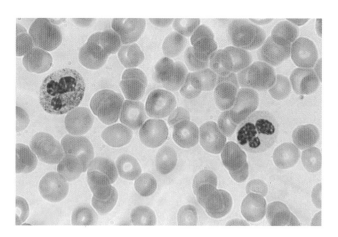

Slide 27. Hypogranular Neutrophil

A decrease in granules within the neutrophils' cytoplasm is most common in the myelodysplastic and myeloproliferative syndromes, reflecting the abnormal cell maturation that is a hallmark of those disorders. Basophils and eosinophils may also be hypogranular. This slide, from a patient with myelodysplasia, demonstrates two neutrophils. The one on the left has cytoplasmic granules; the other is hypogranular.

CYTOPLASMIC INCLUSIONS IN THE NEUTROPHIL

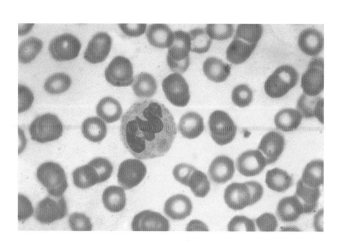

Slide 28. Döhle Bodies

Composed of rough endoplasmic reticulum and glycogen granules, Döhle bodies are single or multiple, small blue-gray inclusions in the cytoplasm of neutrophils, often at the periphery. They may occur in several settings, including uncomplicated pregnancy, infections, inflammatory disorders, burns, myeloproliferative disorders, myelodysplastic syndromes, pernicious anemia, and cancer chemotherapy. The neutrophil in this slide demonstrates a pale, bluish-gray Döhle body in the 5 o'clock position at the edge of the cytoplasm.

IMMATURE NEUTROPHILS AND RED CELLS: LEUKOERYTHROBLASTOSIS

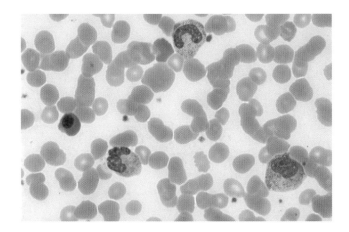

Slide 29. Leukoerythroblastosis

Leukoerythroblastosis is the appearance of nucleated red cells and immature granulocytes on a peripheral smear. The most common cause is the presence in the bone marrow of abnormal cells, which may be excessive hematopoietic stem cells, as in the myelo-dysplastic and myeloproliferative disorders, or malignant cells, as in leukemia or metastatic carcinoma. Other causes include intense bone marrow stimulation because of severe infection, hemolytic anemia, hemorrhage, and megaloblastic anemia. This slide, from a patient with bone marrow metastases, has one nucleated red cell, an early white cell (a myelocyte; see slide 65) near the corner, and two bands.

OTHER GRANULOCYTES

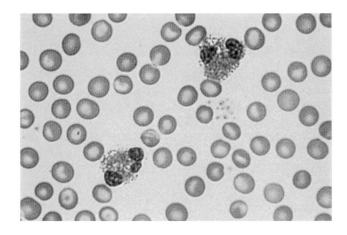

Slide 30. Eosinophil

The eosinophil usually has a bilobed nucleus and heavily condensed chromatin; occasionally a round, single nucleus or one with three lobes is present. The granules, considerably larger than those of neutrophils, are spherical, red-orange, and refractile. They pack the cytoplasm and often overlie the nuclei. Two eosinophils are visible in this slide; one has two lobes, the other has three. The differential diagnosis of eosinophilia is large; the most common causes are allergic diseases, such as asthma and eczema; drug reactions; and parasitic infestations in which the organism, typically a worm, has a stage of tissue invasion. In the center of this slide is a clump of aggregated platelets, an artifact from the anticoagulant present in the tube of collected blood (see discussion of thrombocytopenia on p. 23).

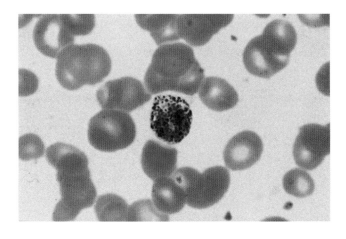

Slide 31. Basophil

Throughout its cytoplasm, the basophil has numerous dark purple granules that typically overlie and obscure the nucleus, which usually has three clover-leaf lobes. In this slide the prominent violaceous granules cover the nucleus, making it impossible to enumerate the lobes. Basophils are characteristically increased in the myeloproliferative disorders, especially in chronic granulocytic leukemia.

MACROPHAGES

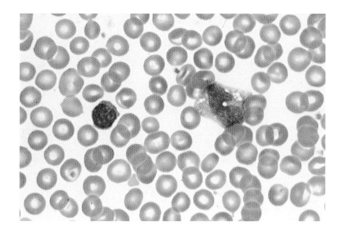

Slide 32. Monocyte

Monocytes, the largest circulating cells normally found in the peripheral blood, measure about 12–20 μm in diameter. They are round, but some have blunt projections (pseudopods) that may indent neighboring cells. The large nucleus is notched, folded, or lobulated and has loose, lacy chromatin strands. The cytoplasm is dull gray-blue and contains numerous, diffuse, usually small and light-colored granules that range from light gray to pink. They may give the cytoplasm a dustlike or ground-glass appearance. Cytoplasmic vacuoles are common. This slide allows comparison of the large, vacuolated monocyte with the surrounding red cells and the small lymphocyte. Increased numbers of monocytes may occur in several conditions, including chronic infections, such as tuberculosis; chronic inflammatory processes, such as rheumatoid arthritis; neoplasms; and certain leukemias.

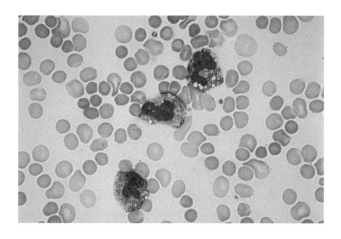

Slide 33. Activated Monocytes

With certain inflammatory conditions, such as bacteremia, the granules of the "activated" monocytes become more prominent. All three monocytes in this slide demonstrate increased granulation. The patient had *Clostridium perfringens* bacteremia complicated by hemolysis, which explains the presence of numerous spherocytes.

LYMPHOCYTES

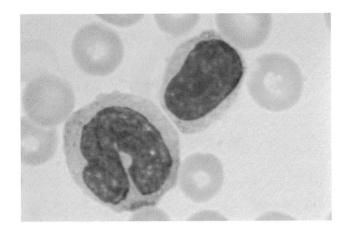

Slide 34. Small Lymphocyte

About 90% of the circulating lymphocytes are small cells (9–12 μm in diameter) with a purplish nucleus approximately 8.5 μm in diameter that contains dense chromatin clumps. A thin rim of cytoplasm devoid of granules surrounds it. About two-thirds of these cells are T-lymphocytes and most of the remainder are B-lymphocytes, but these two types are indistinguishable on routine smears. The smaller cell in this slide is a normal lymphocyte with the typical high nuclear:cytoplasm ratio, closed chromatin, and a very slightly irregular, ovoid nucleus. The larger cell on the left is a monocyte. The causes of increased numbers of lymphocytes are diverse; among the most common are viral infections, adverse drug reactions, and chronic lymphocytic leukemia.

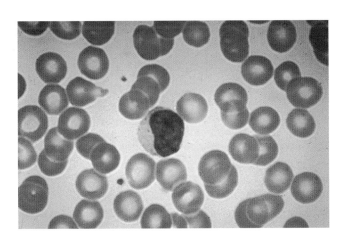

Slide 35. Large Lymphocyte

About 10% of the circulating lymphocytes are larger (12–16 μm in diameter) than the small lymphocytes, have a more abundant cytoplasm, possess a less condensed nuclear chromatin, and often have a more irregular, less rounded shape. In this slide the lymphocyte is much larger than the adjacent normal erythrocytes, the nucleus is large and slightly indented, and the cytoplasm is pale and more abundant than in small lymphocytes.

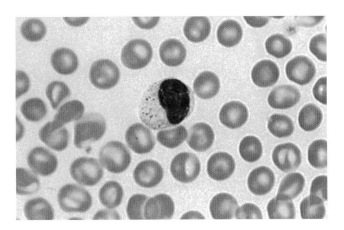

Slide 36. Large Granular Lymphocyte

Some large lymphocytes have several sizable reddish-purple granules in the cytoplasm. Large granular lymphocytes normally constitute about 5% of circulating white cells. Abnormal elevations in large granular lymphocytes may occur in patients with viral infectious, neutropenia, pure red cell aplasia, and rheumatoid arthritis. Often the increase is unexplained, but a leukemia with this cell type can develop. The large granular lymphocyte in this slide harbors several granules in the cytoplasm. Large granular lymphocytes are usually either T cytotoxic/suppressor or natural killer (CNK) cells.

PLASMA CELLS

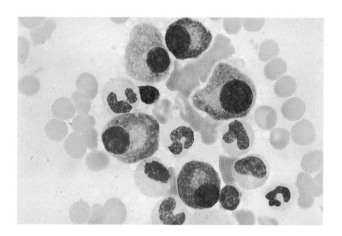

Slide 37. Plasma Cell: Bone Marrow Aspirate

Plasma cells, although ordinarily absent on peripheral smears, may appear with bacterial or viral infections, drug and other allergies, immunizations, and systemic lupus erythematosus. In some patients with multiple myeloma, plasma cells are detectable and initially cytologically normal. They have a diameter of about 14–18 μm, are oval, and possess eccentric nuclei with purple chromatin clumps. The deep blue cytoplasm commonly has vacuoles and is pale near the nucleus (perinuclear clear zone) where the Golgi apparatus is present and immunoglobulins are processed. This slide, taken from a bone marrow aspirate, shows five plasma cells as well as several neutrophil precursors (see later discussion of granulopoiesis).

ABNORMAL MONONUCLEAR CELLS

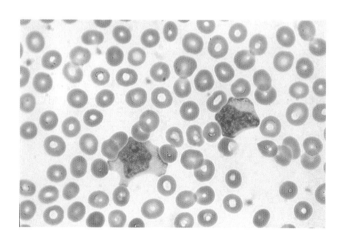

Slide 38. Atypical Lymphocyte

"Atypical" lymphocytes, although diverse in appearance, are usually larger than small lymphocytes and have an oval, kidney-shaped, or lobulated nucleus, which may appear folded. Nucleoli are sometimes prominent, and the chromatin is coarse, reticular, or clumped. The abundant cytoplasm, which often has a deep blue or gray color, lacks granules and is commonly vacuolated or foamy. Where atypical lymphocytes contact red cells, the cytoplasm is frequently indented and the margin more darkly stained. Atypical lymphocytes are most common in viral diseases, especially with Epstein-Barr virus (infectious mononucleosis), but also with cytomegalovirus infection in normal hosts, and occasionally in acute human immunodeficiency virus (HIV) infection. They sometimes occur in drug reactions. In this slide, from a patient with infectious mononucleosis, two large atypical lymphocytes with irregularly shaped nuclei are visible. Both nuclei appear immature in that they have "open" (or reticular) chromatin and one contains a nucleolus. The cytoplasm is basophilic; where the cell borders abut adjacent erythrocytes, the color of the cytoplasm darkens. Taken out of clinical context, these cells could be misinterpreted as circulating blasts in acute leukemia or circulating lymphoma cells, emphasizing the importance of interpreting the hematologic findings in conjunction with the clinical findings.

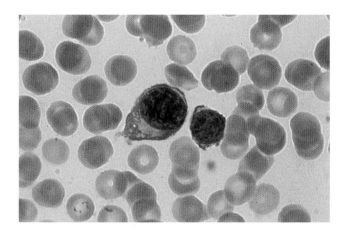

Slide 39. Plasmacytoid Lymphocyte

The plasmacytoid lymphocyte resembles a plasma cell in its dark blue cytoplasm, but the nucleus is less eccentric, the cell is round, and the perinuclear clear space is absent or small. These cells may form in viral infections, lymphomas, multiple myeloma, and Waldenström's macroglobulinemia, the cause of the plasmacytoid lymphocyte, the larger of the two cells, in this slide. It has a dark blue cytoplasm and a small perinuclear clear zone. For comparison, a normal small lymphocyte is present that has less cytoplasm and more condensed nuclear chromatin.

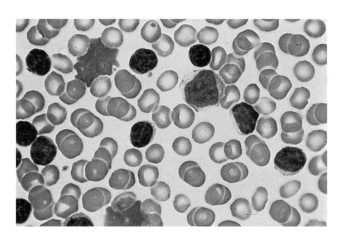

Slide 40. Smudge Cell

Fragile lymphocytes may rupture during the preparation of blood smears, creating smudge cells, in which the nucleus appears spread out, its border hazy, and the cytoplasm meager or absent. This slide reveals two smudge cells, one at top left and one only partially seen at lower left. The patient had chronic lymphocytic leukemia, a condition in which smudge cells sometimes appear in large numbers. The remaining lymphocytes are typical of CLL, except for the large cell with prominent nucleoli, which is a prolymphocyte (see slide 138).

CYTOPLASMIC INCLUSIONS IN MONONUCLEAR CELLS

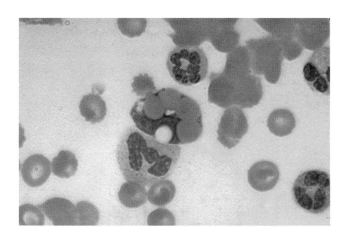

Slide 41. Erythrophagocytosis

Erythrophagocytosis is the presence of intact erythrocytes within the cytoplasm of phagocytic cells. This process may occur in leukemia and with red cell damage from complement-fixing antibody, infectious agents, or chemical poisons. In this slide, from a patient with autoimmune hemolytic anemia, a vacuolated monocyte, hardly recognizable as such, engulfs four erythrocytes. A hypersegmented neutrophil lies above it.

Evaluation of Platelets

Platelet characteristics to evaluate on a blood smear are their number and size, and the presence of granules. Normally the ratio of red cells to platelets is about 10–40:1; approximately 7–20 are present in each oil immersion field when viewed through a 100× objective. Multiplying the number per oil immersion field by 20,000 gives an approximate platelet count per mm³ (μL), or multiplying by 20 gives the count as __ $\times\ 10^9$/L.

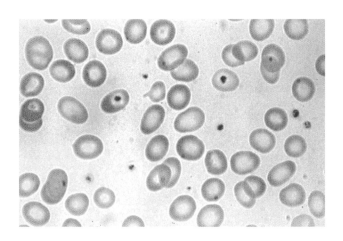

Slide 42. Normal Platelets

Normal platelets are about 1–3 μm in diameter, blue-gray, and contain fine, purple to pink granules that may be diffuse or concentrated in the center of the cells, where they can resemble nuclei. Several platelets are visible in this slide. In the center, platelets overlie two red cells, a situation in which they can mimic erythrocyte inclusions, such as Howell-Jolly bodies or parasites.

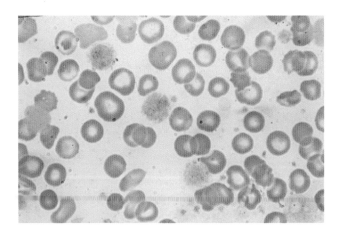

Slide 43. Giant Platelets

Platelets are considered large when about 4–8 μm in diameter and giant when wider (i.e., equal to or larger than a normal erythrocyte). Mean platelet volume (MPV) as measured with an automatic blood cell counter increases when many large platelets are present. Young platelets are usually big. Other causes of large platelets include hereditary conditions, such as Bernard-Soulier syndrome, or acquired disorders, especially immune thrombocytopenia purpura, myeloproliferative disorders, myelodysplasia, disseminated intravascular coagulation, and thrombotic thrombocytopenic purpura. Several giant platelets, replete with granules, are visible in this slide from a patient with chronic granulocytic leukemia. Numerous adjacent normal platelets and red cells permit comparison of their respective sizes.

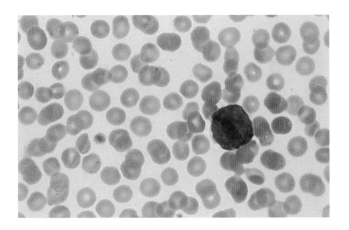

Slide 44. Megakaryocytes

Megakaryocytes are rare in the peripheral blood of normal adults. They usually have little or no cytoplasm. The purplish-red to dark blue nucleus contains dense chromatin and is large, irregularly lobed, and ring- or doughnut-shaped. Megakaryocytes in the peripheral blood are increased in neonates, during pregnancy, in the postpartum period, and after surgery, chest injury, or cardiac massage. They are also seen in myeloproliferative syndromes, infection, and malignancies. The cell in this slide, from a patient with a myeloproliferative disorder, has a large, irregular, violet nucleus with no cytoplasm, characteristic of a circulating megakaryocyte nucleus.

THROMBOCYTOSIS

The normal platelet count in adults is about $150–400 \times 10^9/L$ (150,000–400,000/mm^3), corresponding to about 7–20 per oil immersion field (100× objective). Several conditions may cause thrombocytosis. Movement of platelets from extravascular platelet pools into the intravascular space occurs with epinephrine administration, parturition, and vigorous exercise. Following splenectomy, platelets ordinarily present in the spleen are released into the circulating blood. The resulting thrombocytosis typically resolves, but sometimes only after months to years.

The remaining forms of thrombocytosis arise from increased platelet production rather than from altered distribution. Elevated platelet counts—often to greater than 1 million/mm^3—occur in the myeloproliferative diseases, which

Table 1. Causes of Thrombocytosis

Movement from extravascular pools into circulation
  Splenectomy
  Exercise
  Epinephrine
  Parturition
Myeloproliferative disorders
  Chronic granulocytic leukemia
  Essential thrombocytosis
  Idiopathic myelofibrosis
  Polycythemia vera
Secondary causes
  Iron deficiency anemia
  Malignancy
  Infections
  Noninfectious inflammation
  Acute blood loss
  Hemolysis
  Recovery from thrombocytopenia

are clonal disorders of multipotent stem cells characterized by increased production of one or more of the hematopoietic cell lines. All the myeloproliferative disorders can cause thrombocytosis. These include chronic granulocytic leukemia, polycythemia vera, agnogenic myeloid metaplasia (idiopathic myelofibrosis), and, of course, essential thrombocythemia. The thrombocytosis in these conditions is called "primary."

"Secondary" or "reactive" thrombocytosis develops from other diseases, in many cases probably from cytokines stimulating platelet overproduction. These may arise from infections or from other conditions, such as rheumatoid arthritis, in which inflammation is prominent. Thrombocytosis is common in malignancies, especially lymphomas and cancers of the lung, breast, stomach, colon, and ovary. Acute blood loss, hemolytic anemia, and recovery from thrombocytopenia ("rebound" thrombocytosis) are sometimes associated with increased platelet counts. About 50–75% of patients with iron deficiency anemia have thrombocytosis, especially those with active bleeding. In all of these diseases causing secondary thrombocytosis, the risk of thromboembolic complications is low.

The number of platelets present tends to distinguish among the possible causes of thrombocytosis. With marked thrombocytosis ($>1,000 \times 10^9$/L [$>1,000,000$/mm^3]), the main causes are splenectomy, inflammation or infection, malignancy, and myeloproliferative or other hematologic disorders. When the platelet count exceeds 2 million/mm^3 ($2,000 \times 10^9$/L), the diagnosis is almost certainly a myeloproliferative disease.

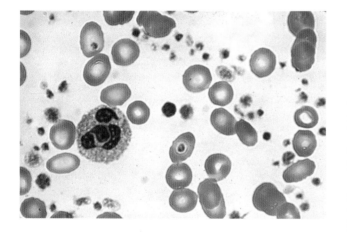

Slide 45. Thrombocytosis

Besides the absolute number of platelets and associated hematologic findings that might suggest a specific diagnosis, the features on the smear that help differentiate the causes of thrombocytosis are the size and appearance of the platelets. Many are large in myeloproliferative disorders and after splenectomy, but they tend to be small in reactive thrombocytosis due to hemorrhage, trauma, iron deficiency, inflammation, infection, and malignancy. In myeloproliferative disorders, hypogranular, agranular, or markedly misshapen platelets may appear. This slide, from a patient with essential thrombocytosis (thrombocythemia), contains numerous platelets that vary in size. Some are large, as expected in a myeloproliferative disorder, and some overlie red cells, mimicking erythrocyte inclusions or parasites.

THROMBOCYTOPENIA

Thrombocytopenia is the presence of fewer than 150,000 platelets/mm^3. Clinical signs related to thrombocytopenia rarely occur until the platelet count is <50,000/mm^3 and become prominent primarily when it is <20,000/mm^3. The findings relate to bleeding into the skin and from mucous membranes. Hemorrhage into the joints and soft tissue, common in hereditary disorders of coagulation such as hemophilia, is rare in thrombocytopenia. The usual cutaneous signs are nonpalpable purpura and petechiae, especially in dependent areas and areas subject to pressure or constriction, such as from the elastic bands of underwear. Bleeding may also be mucosal, including epistaxis and hemorrhage from the genitourinary and gastrointestinal tracts. Petechiae may develop on the dorsum of the tongue, and small hemorrhagic cysts may appear on its ventral surface.

A pseudothrombocytopenia occurs rarely (1 in 1,000 to 1 in 10,000 patients) with blood collected in tubes containing the calcium-chelating anticoagulant EDTA (ethylenediaminetetraacetate). In the presence of this substance, certain antibodies cause platelets to form clumps or to aggregate around neutrophils (satellitism), findings visible on a blood smear. With these physical changes, the automated platelet counters become inaccurate. Employing a different anticoagulant or using nonanticoagulated blood obtained from a fingerstick will usually yield an accurate platelet count.

The causes of genuine thrombocytopenia can be classified into three general groups: (1) inadequate production, (2) increased destruction, and (3) abnormal distribution. Inadequate platelet production can occur from (a) bone marrow hypoplasia caused by such factors as radiation, chemotherapy, or toxins; (b) marrow infiltration by fibrosis, malignancy, or granulomas; (c) selective impairment of platelet production by drugs, infections, or ethanol; (d) ineffective thrombopoiesis because of myelodysplasia or deficiencies in folate or vitamin B$_{12}$; and (e) hereditary diseases such as May-Hegglin anomaly and Wiskott-Aldrich syndrome.

Increased destruction can occur from immune or nonimmune mechanisms. Immune-related thrombocytopenia occurs with (a) systemic lupus erythematosus; (b) lymphoproliferative disorders, such as chronic lymphocytic leukemia; (c) drug reactions, such as to quinidine; (d) infections, such as HIV and infectious mononucleosis; (e) reactions following transfusions; and (f) idiopathic immune thrombocytopenic purpura. Nonimmune causes include (a) severe bleeding; (b) disseminated intravascular coagulation; (c) abnormalities in the small vessels caused by such disorders as vasculitis, thrombotic thrombocytopenic purpura, and hemolytic-uremic syndrome; and (d) infections.

Causes of abnormal distribution include (a) dilutional thrombocytopenia, seen following massive transfusion, and (b) hypersplenism, a condition in

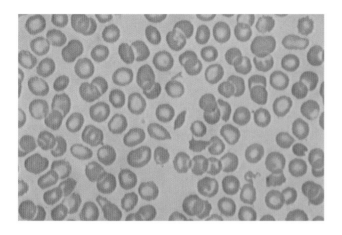

Slide 46. Thrombocytopenia

With thrombocytopenia, fewer than about 7 platelets are visible per oil immersion field with a 100× objective. Associated abnormalities on the blood smear, such as red and white cell aberrations with myelodysplastic syndromes, may suggest the cause, but otherwise the only helpful characteristic is platelet size. In general, platelets are large when thrombocytopenia results from increased destruction and small with diseases of diminished production. In this slide only one platelet is present. The schistocytes indicate that the cause is a microangiopathic process; in this case, the underlying problem was disseminated intravascular coagulation associated with bacterial sepsis.

which cytopenias—anemia, leukopenia, and thrombocytopenia, alone or in any combination—occur as a consequence of splenomegaly. Splenic size is the major determinant of whether hypersplenism occurs; usually the spleen is palpable on examination. The etiology of the splenomegaly is less important, and hypersplenism can develop with spleens enlarged by infections; inflammatory diseases such as systemic lupus erythematosus; congestion from portal hypertension (as with hepatic cirrhosis); neoplasias, benign or malignant; and infiltrative disorders such as sarcoidosis, amyloidosis, and Gaucher's disease. In hypersplenism, the platelet count is usually >50,000/mm³.

Table 2. Causes of Thrombocytopenia

Artifactual	Increased destruction
Platelet clumping with EDTA anticoagulant	Immune related
Inadequate production	Systemic lupus erythematosus
Bone marrow hypoplasia	Lymphoproliferative disorders
Radiation	Drugs
Chemotherapy	Infections
Toxins	Transfusions
Bone marrow infiltration	Idiopathic immune thrombocytopenia
Fibrosis	Nonimmune mechanisms
Malignancy	Severe bleeding
Granulomas	Disseminated intravascular coagulation
Selective impairment of platelet production	Abnormalities in small vessels
Drugs	Vasculitis
Infections	Thrombotic thrombocytopenic purpura
Ethanol	Hemolytic-uremic syndrome
Ineffective thrombopoiesis	Abnormal distribution
Folate or B_{12} deficiency	Dilutional, from massive transfusion
Hereditary disorders	Hypersplenism
May-Hegglin anomaly	
Wiskott-Aldrich syndrome	

Artifacts on Peripheral Smears

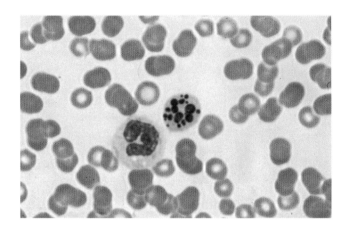

Slide 47. Prolonged Storage

If a substantial delay occurs between the blood collection and smear preparation, the cell morphology may change as the specimen remains in the tube. Excessive heat, dilution of the blood by intravenous fluids, or shaking the specimen also produces artifacts. The subsequent smear can show erythrocyte crenation—the development of spikelike projections on the red cell membrane—and degeneration of the neutrophils' nuclei. In this slide, a band and a neutrophil are present. The neutrophil is shrunken, cytoplasmic granules have disappeared, and its nucleus has broken into numerous condensed fragments. Sometimes these degenerated neutrophils have single or bilobed nuclei and resemble dysplastic cells or nucleated red cells.

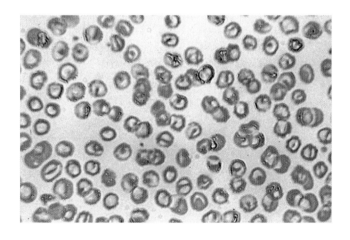

Slide 48. Water Artifact

Water in the methanol solution used in the Wright stain or moisture on the surface of the slide before fixation shrinks and distorts the red cells, making them hypochromic, microcytic, and misshapen, often with crenated borders. Several erythrocytes in this slide resemble target cells. The presence of refractile material in them is the clue to a water artifact, which is present in nearly all the erythrocytes in this slide.

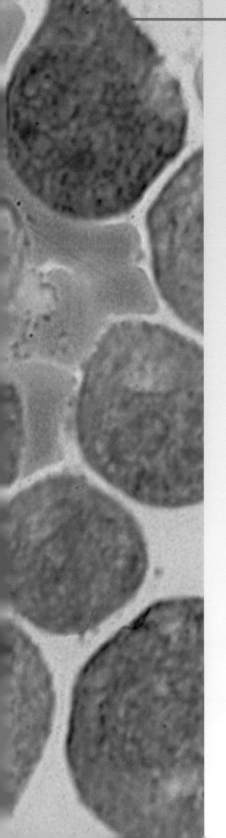

BONE MARROW ASPIRATE

Examination of the Bone Marrow Aspirate

Examination of a bone marrow aspirate should begin at low power, using the 10× objective, to determine whether the specimen contains representative cellular marrow particles that are adequately preserved and stained. The assessment should include a rough estimate of cellularity and megakaryocyte numbers. Using the 20× objective, the examiner should scrutinize the cellular composition, including the myeloid to erythroid (M:E) ratio, the relative numbers of mononuclear versus segmented cells, and the presence of abnormal megakaryocyte forms. At this medium power, the normal aspirate smear should reveal heterogeneous populations of cells, including prominent numbers of maturing members of the myeloid series. A monotonous appearance is definitely abnormal and usually indicates neoplasia. Examination should also include a careful search for metastatic neoplastic cell populations, which may occur in clumps. The cytological detail of individual hematopoietic elements is best evaluated at high power (40× or 50× objective) in areas near stromal fragments where the cells barely touch each other. The observer should scrutinize several hundred cells under high power and determine a differential count to assess pathological increases in subpopulations such as blasts, plasma cells, lymphocytes, eosinophil and basophil precursors, mast cells, and nonhematopoietic cells. In addition, evaluation of erythroid and myeloid precursors should include a search for megaloblastic and dysplastic features. Smears stained for iron require examination under low and high magnification, including oil, to assess storage iron within macrophages and to detect iron granules in erythroid precursors.

Evaluation of the Aspirate

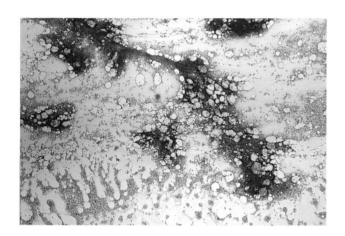

Slide 49. Bone Marrow Aspirate: Low Power

The large dark-staining material represents bone marrow stroma; intermingled with and adjacent to it are bone marrow cells. This combination indicates an adequate sample to examine and one likely to be representative of the marrow as a whole. Areas to evaluate at higher power are those where the cells are well-separated rather than crowded. At this magnification one can enumerate the megakaryocytes and search for nonhematopoietic cell clusters, usually indicative of metastatic malignancy. The vacuoles represent areas of fat dissolved during slide preparation.

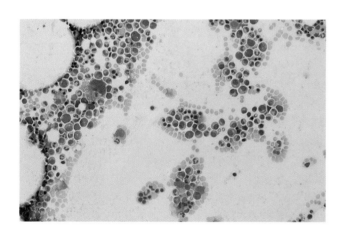

Slide 50. Bone Marrow Aspirate: Medium Power

This slide reveals an appropriate area to examine under medium power: a heterogeneous population of hematopoietic cells, including both myeloid and erythroid precursors, is present, with excellent cytological detail. The cells are well-separated, and the field is near a spicule, which is representative of the marrow. In contrast, substantial numbers of cells distant from spicules often originate from sinusoidal blood and are not representative of the marrow cavity. The largest cell in the field is a megakaryocyte (see slide 69).

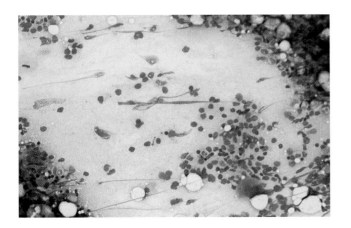

Slide 51. Bone Marrow Aspirate: Artifact

The process of slide preparation may "strip" the cytoplasm from cells, leaving bare nuclei behind. In this slide, the cytoplasm is absent from the cells in the center of the field. This artifact often gives the appearance of increased numbers of monotonous cells, erroneously suggesting malignancy. Because accurately identifying cells is difficult, examination of such areas is misleading.

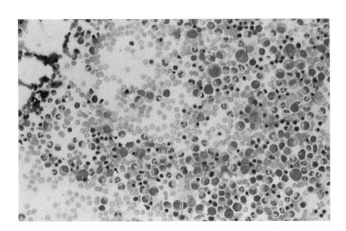

Slide 52. Normal M:E Ratio

Normally, the proportion of myeloid to erythroid precursors (M:E ratio) is about 3:1. In this slide the marrow sample is appropriately cellular, lies near a spicule, has a normal M:E ratio, and demonstrates normal myeloid maturation. The erythroid precursors are small, round cells with closed chromatin, whereas those in the myeloid line are larger, with more cytoplasm. At one edge of the slide is a group of pigment-laden macrophages presumably containing iron, a normal finding (see slide 56).

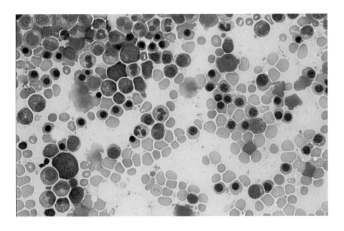

Slide 53. Decreased M:E Ratio

In this slide, the proportion of myeloid precursors is substantially diminished relative to the erythroid series, and the M:E ratio is about 1:1 because of increased erythroid cells. Erythroid hyperplasia can occur as a response to anemia and, less frequently, from neoplastic disorders, such as polycythemia vera.

Iron in the Bone Marrow

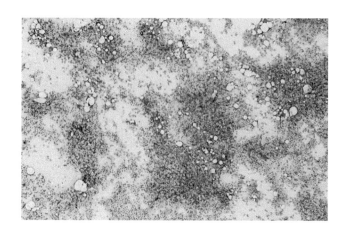

Slide 54. Normal Iron Stores: Prussian Blue Stain

A Prussian blue or Perls' stain delineates hemosiderin in erythroblasts and macrophages as blue-black material. This low-power view of an aspirate discloses a moderate number of stained areas, indicating normal iron in histiocytes, which tend to accumulate in the center of spicules.

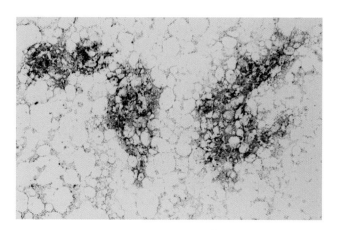

Slide 55. Increased Iron Stores

This sample demonstrates increased amounts of blue-black-staining hemosiderin in bone marrow macrophages. Increased iron stores are common following multiple transfusions and in the anemia of chronic disease, many hemolytic anemias, hemochromatosis, alcoholism, and myelodysplastic disorders. In this case, the cause was iron overload from repeated transfusions.

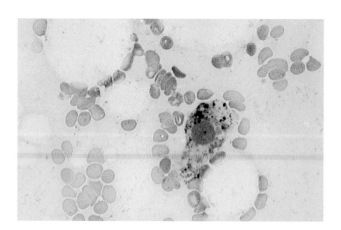

Slide 56. Iron-laden Macrophage

The large cell in this Wright-stained bone marrow aspirate specimen contains numerous dark granules. This appearance suggests iron, an impression that an iron stain can confirm. These cells are normally present in the bone marrow, but a large number of them indicates increased bone marrow iron.

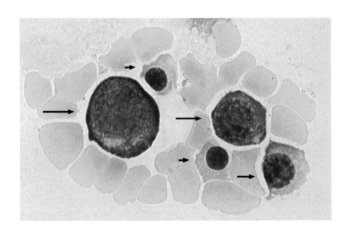

Slide 57. Proerythroblast (Pronormoblast)

The earliest recognizable erythrocyte precursor is a proerythroblast, a round or oval cell about 14–19 μm in diameter. Its large nucleus, which has a regular border, occupies about 80% of the cell and is surrounded by a rim of basophilic cytoplasm, with a characteristic, single perinuclear "hof," an area of clearing that represents the Golgi apparatus. A single prominent nucleolus is typically present, and the nuclear chromatin is red-purple and finely granular or "open." As the erythrocytes mature, the cell size diminishes, the nucleoli disappear, the chromatin condenses, and the color of the cytoplasm changes as red hemoglobin replaces blue-staining RNA. This slide shows the large size of the pronormoblast (*long arrow*), its dark blue cytoplasm, and the fine, diffuse chromatin pattern. Nucleoli are visible in the nucleus. This specimen demonstrates the maturation of red cell precursors, described more completely in subsequent slides. The smaller cell with blue cytoplasm (*medium arrow*) is the basophilic erythroblast. A polychromatophilic erythroblast (*small arrow*) and the two remaining nucleated cells (*tiny arrows*), which are orthochromatic erythroblasts, are also seen. The increasing maturation of the red cells, therefore, is indicated by the decreasing size of the arrows.

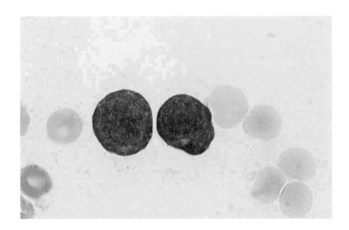

Slide 58. Basophilic Erythroblast

The proerythroblast differentiates into the basophilic erythroblast, a cell about 12–16 μm in diameter, in which nucleoli are absent and the chromatin appears coarse and granular. In this slide the two cells are basophilic erythroblasts. A small perinuclear clear space (hof) lies beneath both nuclei.

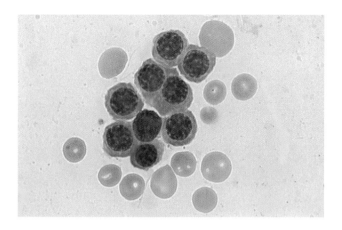

Slide 59. Polychromatophilic Erythroblast

The polychromatophilic erythroblast is 12–15 μm in diameter, and, compared to its predecessor, the basophilic erythroblast, the nucleus is smaller, the chromatin is condensed into irregular clumps, and the cytoplasm is polychromatophilic, that is, blue-gray. Pink areas from hemoglobin may be visible near the nucleus. In this example, a cluster of polychromatophilic erythroblasts appears in the center of the field. The presence of two adjacent polychromatophilic erythrocytes (the large purplish cells) and several mature red cells allows a comparison of their respective diameters.

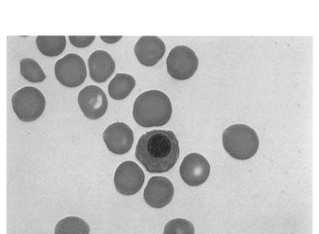

Slide 60. Orthochromatic Erythroblast

The most mature form of the nucleated red cell, the orthochromatic erythroblast, is about 8–12 μm in diameter, contains pink cytoplasm, and has a small nucleus with very condensed chromatin. Compare the size of this orthochromatic erythroblast with the surrounding normal mature red cells. This cell shows some mild nuclear:cytoplasmic dyssynchrony suggestive of megaloblastic changes. The nucleus should be pyknotic (dense and shrunken) at this stage.

ABNORMALITIES IN RED CELL MATURATION

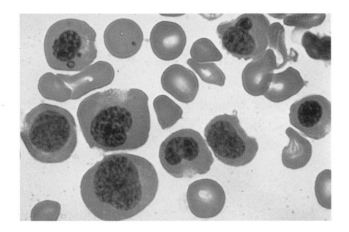

Slide 61. Megaloblastic Anemia

DNA synthesis in the red cell nuclei slows with folate or vitamin B_{12} deficiency or following therapy with drugs that affect DNA synthesis, such as methotrexate and hydroxyurea. The erythrocyte precursors are abnormally large and have more cytoplasm relative to the nucleus than usual. As the cell matures, the chromatin condenses more slowly than normal, and rather than coalescing into a homogeneous mass, demonstrates variable clumping. Because hemoglobin formation is unaffected, the erythrocyte's cytoplasm matures at a normal pace, leading to a so-called nuclear-cytoplasmic dyssynchrony—the nucleus is more primitive than the cytoplasm and has "beaded" chromatin. White cells are also affected: granulocyte precursors are larger than normal and display a similar lack of coordinated nuclear and cytoplasmic maturation. Giant metamyelocytes are especially characteristic, being much larger than normal and often containing a nucleus of unusual shape. Megakaryocytes may be hypersegmented. Hyperplasia of all three hematopoietic lines, especially the erythrocyte precursors, is typically present. In this slide, from a patient with vitamin B_{12} deficiency, the red cell nuclei are too large and the chromatin too dispersed for the degree of cytoplasmic maturation. Howell-Jolly bodies, which may occur with megaloblastic anemias, are present in the two erythrocytes in one corner. With severe megaloblastic changes, dysplastic features may occur, mimicking myelodysplasia. In this slide the irregular nuclear borders and budding are dysplastic findings.

Slide 62. Sideroblastic Anemia: Ringed Sideroblasts, Iron Stain

Normally about 30–50% of erythroblasts contain nonheme iron, visible as a few blue cytoplasmic aggregates on iron stains, such as Prussian blue. These cells are sideroblasts. In a diverse group of erythrocyte maturation disorders characterized by ineffective erythropoiesis and an increased serum iron level, abnormalities in heme synthesis cause an anemia in which sideroblasts containing an increased number of iron granules arranged in an arc or circle around the nucleus appear in the bone marrow. These are ringed sideroblasts. Such sideroblastic anemias may be hereditary or acquired; the latter can occur from ingestion of substances that interfere with pyridoxine metabolism, such as alcohol or drugs, especially isoniazid. An idiopathic form, refractory anemia with ringed sideroblasts, is one of the myelodysplastic syndromes (see slide 122). In sideroblastic anemias, the erythrocytes on the peripheral blood smear may be normochromic and normocytic, but hypochromic, microcytic cells may occur or macrocytic cells may be prominent, and the blood film is sometimes dimorphic, that is, shows two distinct erythrocyte populations. This slide, a Prussian blue stain of a bone marrow aspirate from a patient with myelodysplasia, demonstrates erythroblasts with numerous blue granules that encircle more than one-third of the nucleus, the criterion for a ringed sideroblast.

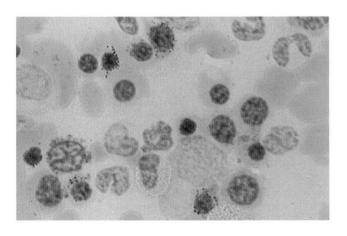

Granulopoiesis

The earliest stages of the neutrophil line, the myeloblast and the promyelocyte, are also the precursors of the eosinophils and basophils. The specific granules allowing differentiation among these three white cell types become distinguishable with the next stage, the myelocyte. The neutrophilic myelocyte matures into the metamyelocyte, which is the immediate predecessor of the band neutrophil. Neutrophils less mature than the band are usually confined to the bone marrow, but they may be present in the peripheral blood in leukemias, in other disorders that disrupt the normal bone marrow architecture, such as myelofibrosis or metastatic malignancy, and sometimes in severe infections.

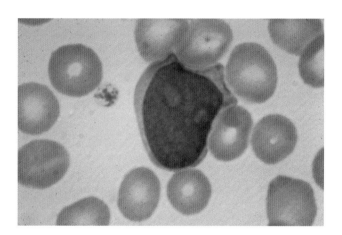

Slide 63. Myeloblast

The most immature cell identifiable as a granulocyte precursor is a myeloblast. About 10–20 μm in diameter, it has a large, reddish-purple, oval or round nucleus with finely dispersed or "open" chromatin and two to five prominent nucleoli. The narrow rim of blue cytoplasm contains no granules. In this slide, three large nucleoli are readily visible. The adjacent red cells, about 8 μm in diameter, permit an estimate of the myeloblast's size.

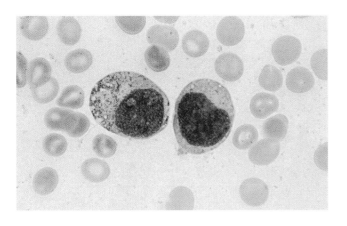

Slide 64. Promyelocyte

The promyelocyte is slightly larger than its predecessor, the myeloblast, and has a somewhat smaller nucleus, typically located eccentrically in the cell and still with two to five nucleoli, a darker blue cytoplasm, and a Golgi zone, a clear area adjacent to the nucleus. The most striking difference from the myeloblast is the presence of reddish-purple, "primary" granules in the cytoplasm. These large granules disappear during maturation, to be replaced by the specific granules that allow distinction among the myeloid cells—neutrophils, basophils, and eosinophils. Aside from the megakaryocyte, the promyelocyte is the largest normal hematopoietic cell in the marrow. This slide demonstrates two promyelocytes, one showing especially well the nucleoli and purplish cytoplasmic granules. The other promyelocyte is more mature, characterized by fewer nucleoli, absent primary granules, and a more central nucleus exhibiting greater clumping of the chromatin.

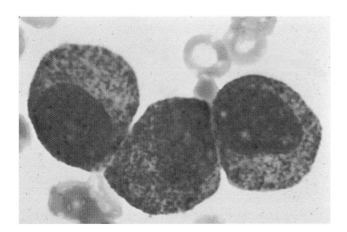

Slide 65. Myelocyte

The myelocyte, smaller than the promyelocyte, often has no nucleoli, possesses a less prominent Golgi zone, and contains granules within its cytoplasm that allow identification of the cell as belonging to the neutrophil, basophil, or eosinophil series. The nucleus is round to slightly oval, and the chromatin shows some coarse clumping. This slide demonstrates three myelocytes of varying maturation, one retaining primary granules, but all having specific granules that are gray and finely dispersed.

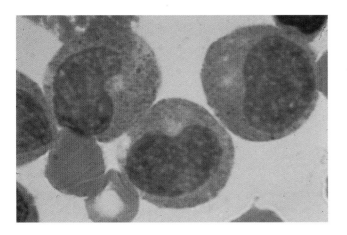

Slide 66. Metamyelocyte

The metamyelocyte, about 10–12 μm in diameter, has an elliptical to horseshoe-shaped nucleus with markedly clumped chromatin and a plentiful, grayish-pink cytoplasm. A metamyelocyte with a U-shaped nucleus differs from the next stage, a band form, whose nucleus is thinner and uniform in width. The three metamyelocytes in this slide reveal the indentation of the nuclei, which show much more chromatin clumping than the myelocytes in the previous slide.

ABNORMALITIES IN WHITE CELL MATURATION

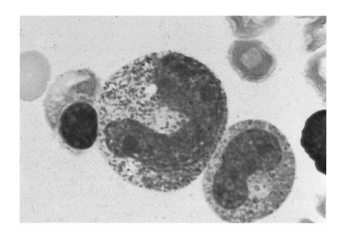

Slide 67. Giant Band

In megaloblastic anemias (see slide 61) the white cells, especially the metamyelocyte, may be larger than normal. Bands can be enlarged as well, as indicated in this slide from a patient with folate deficiency. The normal erythrocyte (measuring about 8 μm in diameter) near the two white cells allows a size comparison. The normal band is approximately 12–15 μm in diameter, the normal metamyelocyte about 10–12 μm.

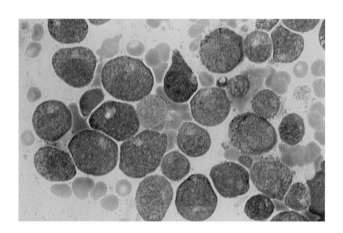

Slide 68. Maturation Arrest

In some situations, including severe congenital neutropenia and agranulocytosis from a chemical or medication, the early white cell precursors are present but the more mature granulocytes are absent. This situation is called "maturation arrest," but it actually represents a left-shifted granulocytic response to injury in the myeloid lineage. In this slide no myelocytes, bands, or mature neutrophils are present. Most of the white cell precursors are promyelocytes.

Thrombopoiesis

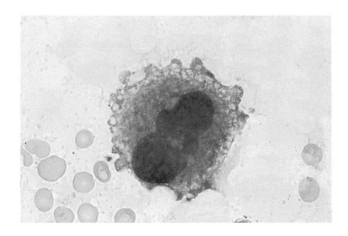

Slide 69. Megakaryocyte

The biggest hematopoietic cell in the bone marrow (30–160 μm), the megakaryocyte has a large nucleus with multiple but contiguous lobes and a basophilic, finely granular cytoplasm ranging from sparse to abundant, depending on the cell's maturity. The margins are irregular, often showing platelets budding off the cytoplasm, which may contain azurophilic granules. This slide demonstrates a megakaryocyte with a multilobulated nucleus and a finely granular cytoplasm with knobby borders, representing young platelets emerging from the megakaryocyte.

ABNORMALITIES IN PLATELET MATURATION

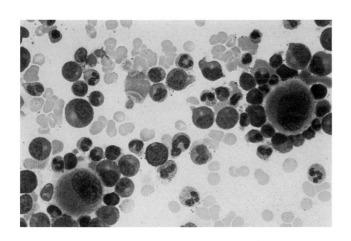

Slide 70. Small Megakaryocyte

Frequently in myelodysplastic syndromes and occasionally in myeloproliferative disorders, megakaryocytes are small, with a decrease in both the size of the nucleus and the cytoplasm, which has poor granulation. This slide, from a patient with chronic granulocytic leukemia, demonstrates two small megakaryocytes in opposite corners. Granulocytic hyperplasia is present, but maturation is normal, as evidenced by numerous mature neutrophils.

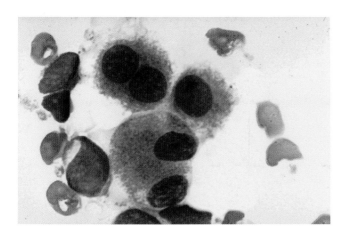

Slide 71. Dysplastic Megakaryocytes

In myelodysplastic disorders, several abnormalities in the megakaryocytes may occur. They may be small (see slide 70), and their nuclei may demonstrate decreased lobulation, bizarre shapes, and the presence of several separate, rather than contiguous, lobules. This slide, from a patient with myelodysplasia, reveals three abnormal megakaryocytes, one with a single nucleus and two containing clearly separated nuclear lobules. The smallest megakaryocyte is a micromegakaryocyte, characteristically equal in size to or smaller than a promyelocyte.

Other Cells in the Bone Marrow Aspirate

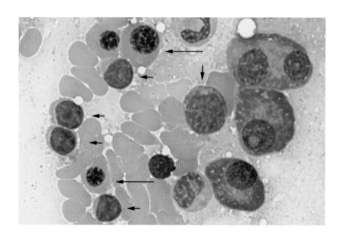

Slide 72. Lymphocyte

In normal adults, lymphocytes constitute up to 20% of the nucleated cells in the bone marrow. They appear as small cells with a rounded or slightly indented nuclei, surrounded by a thin rim of light blue cytoplasm. In this slide, *short horizontal arrows* identify four lymphocytes. Three late erythroid precursors in this smear allow comparison between these cells and the lymphocytes. The erythroid precursors (*long horizontal arrows*) have more abundant cytoplasm, and their nuclei are rounder, with more regular borders, and a more clumped chromatin. This slide also demonstrates some abnormal cells: three atypical plasma cells with prominent nucleoli (one with two nuclei), and a plasmacytoid lymphocyte (*vertical arrow*). The patient had Waldenström's macroglobulinemia (see slide 159).

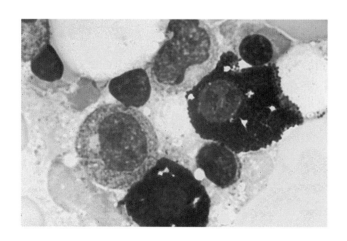

Slide 73. Mast Cell

Mast cells, normally present in the marrow, range from about 5 to 25 μm in diameter. They contain numerous purple granules that do not totally obscure the nucleus, as they often do in basophils. Furthermore, the nucleus is not lobulated, as it is in basophils, and the chromatin is not so clumped. Bone marrow mast cells are increased in lymphoproliferative disorders, such as lymphomas and Waldenström's macroglobulinemia, in myeloproliferative and myelodysplastic syndromes, in chronic liver and renal diseases, and in systemic mast cell disease, a neoplastic process that may range from an indolent disorder to a leukemic form. This slide demonstrates two mast cells. See also slides 187 and 188.

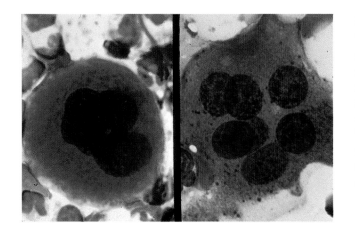

Slide 74. Osteoclasts

This composite slide compares an osteoclast on the right with a megakaryocyte on the left. The osteoclast is involved in bone resorption. It is a large cell, ranging in diameter from 20 to 150 μm, with separate, multiple, round to oval nuclei of uniform size. Reddish granules are present throughout its abundant bluish cytoplasm. In contrast to osteoclasts, normal megakaryocytes have single nuclei that are lobulated and contiguous, not multiple separate nuclei. Their cytoplasm does not contain reddish granules.

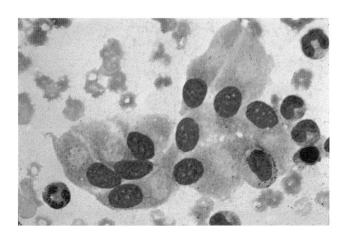

Slide 75. Osteoblasts

Osteoblasts form new bone. They are uncommon in adult bone marrow specimens, where they may appear in small clusters. They occur in areas of bone remodeling following injury, such as fractures or metastatic malignancy. They may mimic metastatic foci or plasma cells because they resemble epithelial cells and tend to form cohesive clumps. They have oval, eccentric nuclei with clumped chromatin. The nuclei may appear to extend beyond the border of the abundant blue-gray cytoplasm, which has a clear area (Golgi region) that is not directly adjacent to the nucleus, as it is in plasma cells. This slide depicts a cohesive group of osteoblasts.

Abnormalities in Cell Type or Number

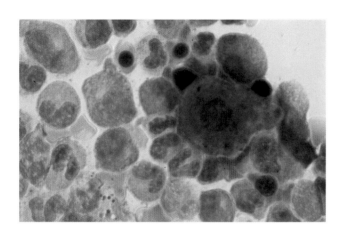

Slide 76. Sea-Blue Histiocyte

Sea-blue histiocytes are bone marrow macrophages with small nuclei and an enormous, often coarse, blue-green cytoplasm. They occur in diseases with high turnover of bone marrow cells because the macrophages ingest the lipids released during cell death. Examples include the myeloproliferative states, especially chronic granulocytic leukemia; myelodysplasia; thalassemia; sickle cell anemia; and immune thrombocytopenia purpura. They are also present in Niemann-Pick disease, in which an enzyme defect causes excessive accumulation of phospholipids, predominantly sphingomyelin, which bone marrow histiocytes consume. The large cell in the right central area of this slide demonstrates the size of the sea-blue histiocyte and its coarse aquamarine cytoplasm. The patient had chronic granulocytic leukemia, and granulocytic hyperplasia is present.

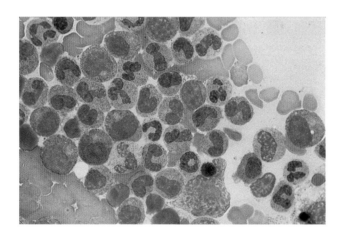

Slide 77. Granulocytic Hyperplasia

Ordinarily, the ratio of myeloid to erythroid precursors is about 3–5:1. In some conditions, including sustained infection, chronic inflammation, leukemia, and response to certain drugs, the number of granulocytes increases. In this slide, from a patient with chronic granulocytic leukemia, virtually all the cells are myeloid, but maturation is normal.

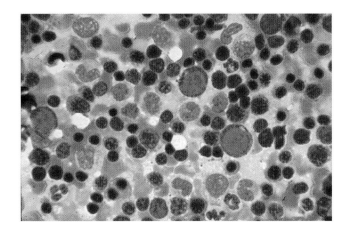

Slide 78. Erythroid Hyperplasia

In several situations, including hemolytic anemia, hemorrhage, and chronic hypoxemia, the number of erythroid precursors increases, but cellular maturation and morphology remain normal. In this slide, from a patient who had a severe hemorrhage, the usual myeloid-to-erythroid ratio is reversed, there being about three times as many erythrocytes as white cells.

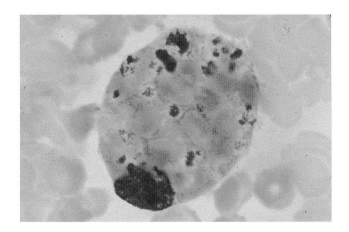

Slide 79. Hemophagocytosis

Various disorders can provoke an increase in histiocytes that ingest numerous bone marrow cells. The most common causes have been infections, especially with the herpesviruses, including Epstein-Barr virus, *Herpes simplex,* and cytomegalovirus. It may occur in patients with AIDS. Other infectious causes include bacteria, especially gram-negative bacilli; fungi; mycobacteria; and rickettsiae. Usually, pancytopenia is present in the peripheral blood, and the bone marrow shows increased benign-appearing macrophages replete with various cells. A familial form also occurs. In addition, hemophagocytosis may develop in certain cancers, especially lymphomas, in which either the ingesting cells or neighboring ones have malignant characteristics. In this slide, from a patient with infection-induced hemophagocytosis, both red cells and platelets stuff the macrophage's cytoplasm.

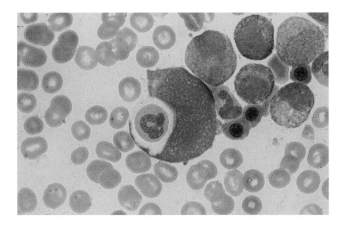

Slide 80. Emperipolesis

Sometimes a cell enters another cell without being destroyed. This event can occur in the marrow when various cells, including platelets, leukocytes, and erythrocytes, move into megakaryocytes. This phenomenon is most common in blood loss, hemolytic anemias, and several neoplasms. In this slide, a megakaryocyte contains a granulocyte.

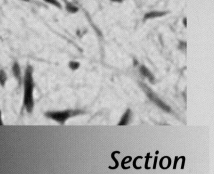

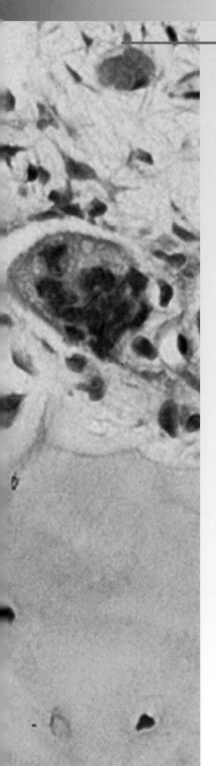

BONE MARROW BIOPSY

Examination of Bone Marrow Biopsy Sections

Whereas the aspirate smear reveals fine cytological details and thus provides information about the maturation and lineage of individual hematopoietic cells, biopsy specimens demonstrate overall cellularity and marrow architecture. The examiner should view the entire section at low power, preferably with a 4× objective, to evaluate changes in the bony trabeculae and marrow elements. Structural abnormalities detectable at low power include metastatic foci, granulomas, lymphomatous aggregates, necrosis, amyloid deposition, and fibrosis. At this magnification, one can also determine the location of immature myeloid precursors relative to the bony trabeculae and the degree of maturation. Medium-power examination of the specimen permits enumeration of megakaryocytes and an assessment of the relative proportions of myeloid and erythroid precursors.

Special histochemical or immunochemical studies can be performed on biopsy sections. Histochemical stains, for example, may demonstrate infectious organisms such as fungi and acid-fast bacilli or help quantify the degree of reticulin fibrosis present. Immunohistochemical stains help to determine phenotypes of abnormal cells in the marrow cavity and are indispensable in discerning whether an abnormal cellular infiltrate derives from marrow or represents metastatic malignancy. In addition, immunohistochemical studies assist in elucidating whether abnormal B-cell lymphoid cell populations, including plasma cells, are clonal.

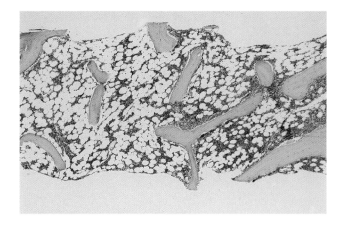

Slide 81. Bone Marrow Biopsy: Low Power

This slide shows several bony trabeculae (the homogeneous, pink-staining sections), which are normally thin, as here. The cellular portions of the marrow contain the hematopoietic cells, and the clear spaces represent areas where fat has dissolved during slide preparation. At birth, bone marrow specimens normally show nearly complete cellularity, with very few fat cells. With age, the cellularity diminishes, and the amount of fat increases. This low-power view allows an estimate of marrow cellularity, which can be expressed as the percentage of the space between trabeculae occupied by cells. In this case, the estimated cellularity is 30%, the expected amount for an older adult.

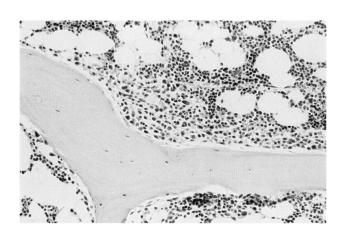

Slide 82. Bone Marrow Biopsy: Medium Power

This slide of normal bone marrow shows a trabecula at medium power, disclosing the presence of clear spaces (lacunae) in which osteocytes reside. The cellularity is normal and comprises a heterogeneous population of myeloid and erythroid precursors. The immature myeloid precursors are characteristically present next to the trabeculae ("paratrabecular").

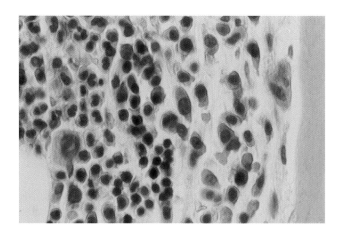

Slide 83. Bone Marrow Biopsy: High Power

This specimen discloses a trabecula bordering the right edge of the slide. Adjacent to it are spindle-shaped cells, osteoblasts, and a large multinucleated cell, likely an osteoclast. Ordinarily, as here, the next zone contains immature myeloid precursors, which are large cells with eosinophilic cytoplasm and a medium nuclear:cytoplasm ratio. Normally, a further step away from the trabecula lie the erythroid precursors, characterized by round, regular, and central nuclei containing closed chromatin and meager or no cytoplasm. This normal arrangement of cells is reversed in myelodysplasia, where myeloid precursors are isolated in islands away from their normal paratrabecular location, a situation known as abnormal localization of immature precursors (ALIP).

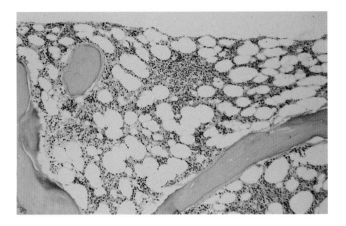

Slide 84. Benign Lymphoid Aggregate

These aggregates, which contain small, mature lymphocytes, sometimes accompanied by plasma cells, are common in bone marrow biopsies, especially in older people. They are usually sparse and well-delineated areas distant from the trabeculae. They may be numerous in various inflammatory and infectious diseases, myeloproliferative disorders, and lymphomas. In this slide a small lymphoid aggregate is visible in the upper central area as an isolated, round collection of cells between bony trabeculae.

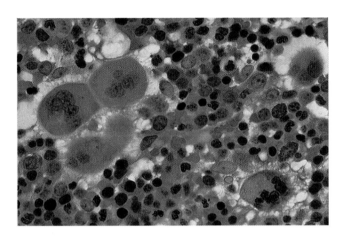

Slide 85. Megakaryocytes

Megakaryocytes are usually obvious on bone marrow biopsies as large cells with multilobed nuclei and a fine, granular cytoplasm. They ordinarily occur away from the trabeculae and are present alone or in clumps of a few cells. In this slide, the five large cells are megakaryocytes; three lie in a cluster. Erythroid hyperplasia is also present in this patient with polycythemia vera.

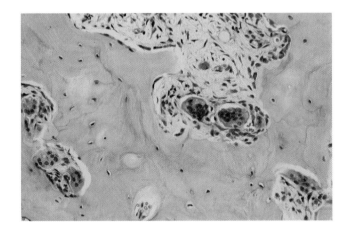

Slide 86. Bone Marrow Osteocytes, Osteoclasts, and Osteoblasts

The osteocytes reside within the small lacunae of the trabeculae. The large multinucleated cells in this slide are osteoclasts. Lining up against the trabeculae are the osteoblasts, which are mononuclear cells with an eccentric nucleus and a prominent Golgi zone. They are best seen in the large marrow space, void of hematopoietic cells, lining the trabecula in a layer of single cells. This area also demonstrates a proliferation of fibroblasts indicative of fibrosis. In this case of Paget's disease, the thick, irregular bony trabeculae have a whorled appearance. The haphazard nature of the increased osteoid can produce a mosaic appearance, characteristic of this disorder. Thickened trabeculae may also occur in chronic renal failure, idiopathic myelofibrosis, systemic mast cell disease, and osteoblastic metastatic malignancy, primarily from prostate or breast cancers.

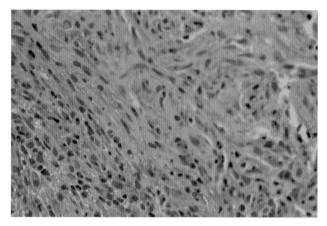

Slide 87. Fibrosis

Bone marrow fibrosis refers to an increase in reticulin, collagen, or both, produced by fibroblasts, which are normally present in the marrow. Reticulin is best identified on silver stains (see next slide), while trichrome stains delineate collagen. A fine pattern of reticulin is normal in the bone marrow, but collagen is not. Fibrosis is a common reaction in many neoplasms, including chronic myeloproliferative disorders, various leukemias, mast cell disease, and metastatic malignancies. It may also develop from radiation treatment, chemotherapy, and exposure to certain toxins. It appears as amorphous material, in which the fibroblasts, with their elongated purplish nuclei, may be numerous or relatively sparse. The orientation of these nuclei sometimes creates a pattern of whorls. This slide, from a patient with idiopathic myelofibrosis, demonstrates a large number of fibroblasts, which are the spindle-shaped cells; in the upper portion they create a swirling appearance. On the left, single cells line up in a row ("Indian file"), another sign of fibrosis.

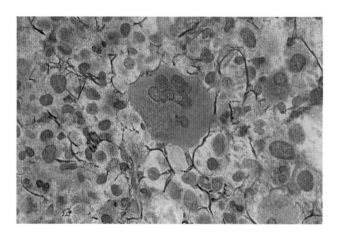

Slide 88. Reticulin Fibrosis

On silver stains of normal bone marrow, a fine, sparse network of reticulin surrounds blood vessels. Manifestations of increased reticulin include thickening of the existing reticulin, more diffuse involvement of the bone marrow, and encirclement of individual hematopoietic cells. Increased reticulin fibrosis often portends a poor prognosis in myelodysplastic and myeloproliferative disorders. This slide, a silver stained–specimen from a patient with polycythemia vera, demonstrates a central megakaryocyte and a pattern of reticulin that is both coarser and more extensive than normal.

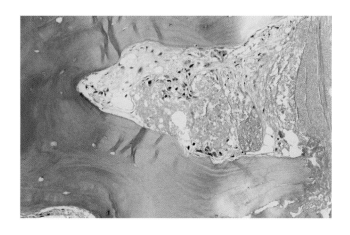

Slide 89. Bone Marrow Necrosis

Extensive death of bone marrow cells may occur from ischemia or increased levels of cytokines, such as tumor necrosis factor. Many patients have fever and bone pain. With extensive marrow involvement, pancytopenia may develop and leukoerythroblastosis appear on the peripheral blood smear. Causes include sickle cell anemia, leukemias, lymphomas, metastatic carcinomas, disseminated intravascular coagulation, and various infections, such as gram-negative bacteremia, miliary tuberculosis, and systemic fungal disease. Early on, the cell borders become indistinct ("ghost cells"), and the nuclei show condensation and irregular margins. Later, the outlines between cells disappear, replaced by an amorphous granular eosinophilic debris, with nuclei either markedly abnormal or absent. In this slide, much of the specimen exhibits amorphous pink granular material; where nuclei are visible, the cell outlines are blurred. Several empty lacunae in the trabeculae indicate that necrosis involved both the bone and the marrow.

Slide 90. Bone Marrow Granuloma

Granulomas are aggregates of altered macrophages called epithelioid cells, accompanied by various combinations of other cells, including fibroblasts, lymphocytes, plasma cells, neutrophils, and eosinophils. The epithelioid histiocytes have abundant pink cytoplasm and large nuclei with dispersed chromatin. When several of these cells coalesce, they form giant cells, which may be of two kinds: the Langhans type, with the nuclei positioned in the periphery of the cell, or the Touton type, with the nuclei dispersed throughout the cell. The most common cause of granulomas is an infection, especially mycobacterial or fungal, but many other organisms can produce the same tissue reaction, including rickettsiae, gram-negative bacilli (e.g., typhoid fever and tularemia), and herpesviruses. The most common noninfectious causes are sarcoidosis, lymphomas, nonhematologic malignancies, and various medications. Sometimes caseation necrosis, defined as the presence of pink granular material in the center of the granuloma, occurs. Usually this pattern indicates an infectious cause, primarily mycobacteria or fungi, and its presence warrants special stains to detect microorganisms. In this slide, from a patient with HIV infection and tuberculosis, an aggregate of epithelioid histiocytes, fibroblasts, and scattered lymphocytes lies in the center. In immunocompromised patients, the granulomas are often poorly delineated, and infections with organisms like mycobacteria may elicit only an increased number of histiocytes that are diffusely distributed or aggregated into loose collections.

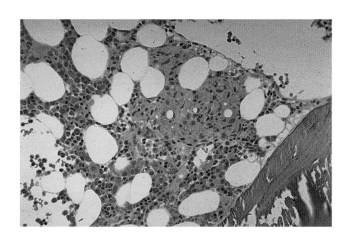

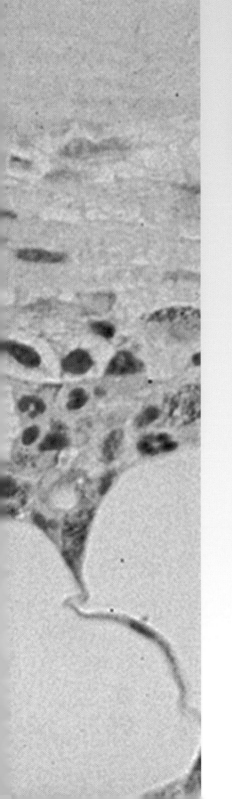

Section 4

SPECIFIC DISORDERS

Anemias

ANEMIA: GENERAL CONSIDERATIONS

Anemia is an abnormally low number of circulating erythrocytes. The World Health Organization (WHO) has defined anemia in adults as a hemoglobin <13 g/dL in males and <12 g/dL in females. Corresponding hematocrits are <39 and <36, respectively. The normal hemoglobin values for blacks in the United States are about 0.5 g/dL less. Although the elderly are more frequently anemic by WHO standards than younger adults, the diminished red cell mass seems to reflect an increased prevalence of disease rather than a normal manifestation of aging. Accordingly, the same values for defining anemia apply to adults of all ages.

Patients often have no symptoms or signs attributable to anemia, especially when it is mild and gradual in onset. When complaints occur, fatigue and lack of energy are common. With severe anemias, dyspnea may develop because of the decreased oxygen-carrying capacity of the blood or because of high-output congestive heart failure, which rarely occurs with hematocrits >20 in the absence of other cardiac disease. Tachycardia and increased force of ventricular contraction may cause palpitations, and the combination of greater flow rate, lowered blood viscosity, and increased turbulence can produce cardiac ("flow") murmurs, characteristically systolic and most commonly in the pulmonic area. In patients with coronary artery disease, angina may worsen because diminished oxygen delivery augments myocardial ischemia. The more rapid velocity of blood through the cranial arteries may cause a whirring sensation in the head. Neurologic symptoms sometimes present in severe anemia include dizziness, faintness, headache, and decreased concentration. Pallor in the conjunctiva, face, or palms suggests anemia, especially when present in all three sites. In severe anemia, retinal hemorrhages can occur. They are often diffuse and are typically flame-shaped or round. Sometimes the hemorrhages have white centers (Roth's spots). Other funduscopic findings include tortuous veins; cotton-wool spots, representing infarction of the retinal nerve cell layer; preretinal hemorrhages; and hard exudates, which are extravasations of proteinaceous material from leaky vessels.

Anemia is not a diagnosis itself but a manifestation of an underlying disease, and its physiologic effects vary from individual to individual. The numerous causes of anemia are diverse; generally, two different systems have been used to classify them. One is by red cell morphology, the other by pathophysiology (or red cell kinetics). Each classification has three major subsets. The morphologic system divides anemias into (1) microcytic (MCV < 80), hypochromic (MCH < 30); (2) macrocytic (MCV > 100), normochromic (MCH 30–34); and (3) normocytic (MCV 80–100), normochromic. With some disorders, the size of the red cell is quite variable, and therefore the same disease may be classified in more than one category, depending on the individual patient. For example, in the anemia of chronic disease the red cells may be either normocytic or microcytic, and in hypothyroidism they are sometimes macrocytic and sometimes normocytic.

Microcytic, hypochromic anemias are disorders of hemoglobin synthesis with impairments resulting from inadequate iron, abnormal globin formation, or the deficiencies in porphyrin and heme synthesis that occur in sideroblastic anemia. The most common cause of microcytic anemias is iron deficiency, usually from blood loss. Microcytosis occurs in about 20% of patients with anemia of chronic disease, in which part of the pathophysiology is impaired transfer of iron to the plasma from its site of storage in macrophages. Examples of impaired globin synthesis leading to microcytosis are the thalassemias and certain hemoglobinopathies, such as hemoglobin C and E. Sideroblastic anemias causing microcytosis include those resulting from lead poisoning and pyridoxine deficiency.

Macrocytic anemias may arise from abnormal DNA synthesis, producing megaloblastic changes in the bone marrow. The major causes include deficiencies in vitamin B_{12} and folate. Macrocytic anemias may also occur from other mechanisms. With recent hemorrhage and with hemolytic anemias, red cells leave the bone marrow at an earlier stage of development than normal, when they are larger than the usual circulating erythrocytes. These cells may still contain a nucleus or, more commonly, have some residual RNA, which stains blue, along with the hemoglobin, which stains red. The result is a purple cell that is larger than normal and is called a polychromatophilic ("lover of many colors") or polychromatic ("many-colored") erythrocyte (see slide 19). When a large number of these cells are present, the MCV can exceed 100. Another common cause of macrocytosis is alcoholism, even in the absence of folate or vitamin B_{12} deficiency, apparently from a direct effect of ethanol on the bone marrow. Usually, however, anemia is absent. Hypothyroidism, through unknown mechanisms, can cause a mild macrocytic anemia. In myelodysplasia, a disease primarily of the elderly, abnormal maturation of red cell precursors often produces macrocytosis.

Normocytic, normochromic anemias arise from several heterogeneous disorders. With hemorrhage or hemolysis the bone marrow may respond appropriately by increasing the number of early red cells. In the other forms of normocytic, normochromic anemia an inadequate bone marrow response occurs because of intrinsic bone marrow disease, diminished erythropoietin, or insufficient iron. *Intrinsic bone marrow disease* includes (1) hypoplasia, such as in aplastic anemia or pure red cell aplasia; (2) infiltration by abnormal tissue, as in multiple myeloma, leukemia, fibrosis, or metastatic malignancy; and (3) myelodysplastic disorders, in which abnormal maturation occurs. *Decreased erythropoietin* can occur from (1) an impaired source, namely renal failure; (2) reduced stimulation, thought to be the cause of anemia in various endocrine disorders, such as hypothyroidism and testosterone deficiency; and (3) interference with its production by inflammatory cytokines, probably a significant component in the pathogenesis of the anemia of chronic disease. In that disorder, other mechanisms include a slight decrease in red cell life span and diminished proliferation of erythroid progenitor cells, also attributed to the effect of inflammatory cytokines. *Insufficient iron* may be a minor element in the pathogenesis of the anemia of chronic disease as well, since the serum iron level is low despite adequate stores in the bone marrow. Early iron deficiency anemia is often normocytic, but as its severity increases, the red cell size diminishes.

A useful laboratory test in evaluating anemias is the reticulocyte count, which enumerates the number of immature red cells that still contain residual RNA. The tests for reticulocyte count involve mixing red cells with a dye, such as brilliant cresyl blue, which will stain the precipitated RNA, and counting the number of erythrocytes with blue granules or reticulum among 1,000 red cells. Automated methods utilize a chemical, such as thiazole orange, which binds to RNA and fluoresces, identifying these young cells. The count is expressed as a percentage—the number of reticulocytes per 100 erythrocytes—or in absolute numbers per volume. The use of the reticulocyte percentage requires a correction for the severity of anemia, which is done by multiplying the percentage by the patient's hemoglobin (or hematocrit) divided by the normal hemoglobin (hematocrit). For example, if the initial reticulocyte count is 4% and the patient's hematocrit is 25, the corrected value is $4\% \times (25/45) = 2.2\%$. A further correction is necessary if the anemia is severe and polychromasia is present on the peripheral blood smear. Ordinarily, the polychromatophilia of immature red cells lasts 4 days, 3 of which are spent in the bone marrow. When these cells are released early, the blue color may last for 2 or even 3 days in the circulating blood. For the reticulocyte percentage to reflect actual red cell production, it should be divided by 2 if the hematocrit is 25 or lower when polychromatophilia is prominent. The reticulocyte percentage after these corrections is called the reticulocyte index. The absolute reticulocyte count or the reticulocyte index is especially useful in distinguishing among the normocytic, normochromic anemias. Anemias with low reticulocyte counts occur from either decreased erythropoietin levels or impaired bone marrow response, and those with elevated reticulocyte counts have increased erythrocyte production in response to hemorrhage or hemolysis.

The reticulocyte count is an important element in the classification of anemias by red cell kinetics. In this scheme, anemias are (1) hypoproliferative, in which the bone marrow cannot increase its red cell production; (2) maturation disorders, in which bone marrow erythroid hyperplasia occurs, but because of defects in cytoplasmic or nuclear maturation, many red cells die in the bone marrow, a situation labeled ineffective erythropoiesis; or (3) hemolysis, in which erythroid hyperplasia occurs and intact red cells leave the bone marrow but are prematurely destroyed in the peripheral circulation. To categorize an anemia, red cell production is determined by the reticulocyte index and a bone marrow sample. In the absence of anemia, the reticulocyte index is normally 1. With moderately severe anemia and a normal bone marrow response, the reticulocyte index should exceed 3. In a bone marrow sample of a patient without anemia the normal erythroid:myeloid (E:M) ratio is 1:3. The expected response to moderately severe anemia is an erythroid hyperplasia that increases that ratio to >1:1. Measuring serum levels of indirect bilirubin and LDH help determine the presence of red cell destruction. These levels should increase whether the erythrocytes are destroyed in the bone marrow or in the peripheral circulation. As with the classification by red cell morphology, some anemias may have characteristics of more than one category. In the anemia of renal disease, for example, the mechanisms responsible include both hypoproliferation, because of decreased erythropoietin levels, and hemolysis, because red cell life span diminishes in a uremic environment. When more than one pathogenic element is present, the anemia is categorized by the predominant mechanism.

In hypoproliferative anemias the red cells are usually normocytic, normochromic, the reticulocyte index is <2, the E:M ratio is <1:2, and the indirect bilirubin is normal or low. Early iron deficiency anemia and the anemia of chronic disease are hypoproliferative. Other causes include decreased erythropoietin secretion (renal failure) or response (endocrine disorders, such as hypothyroidism), and bone marrow damage involving the stem cells (e.g., chemotherapy, aplastic anemia) or marrow structure (metastatic malignancies, myelofibrosis), or through autoimmune or unknown mechanisms (e.g., pure red cell aplasia, systemic lupus erythematosus). Polychromasia, reflecting erythropoietin stimulus, is present in marrow damage and iron deficiency, but absent or diminished with renal failure and inflammation.

With anemias from nuclear or cytoplasmic maturation disorders, the reticulocyte index is <2, the E:M ratio is >1:1 when the anemia is severe, and the indirect bilirubin and LDH levels are increased, except in iron deficiency anemia. Polychromasia, representing erythropoietin stimulation, is present. In cytoplasmic disorders, defective hemoglobin production results in microcytic red cells. Examples are severe iron deficiency, the thalassemias, sideroblastic anemias, and some hemoglobinopathies. In nuclear maturation disorders the red cells are macrocytic, and the primary diseases are deficiencies in vitamin B_{12} and folic acid.

The other major cause of anemia is increased loss or destruction; blood loss usually accounts for the former and hemolysis the latter. In hemolytic anemias the red cells are normocytic or macrocytic (depending on the number of large, immature erythrocytes present), polychromasia is prominent, the reticulocyte index is >3, the E:M ratio is >1:1, and serum LDH and indirect bilirubin levels are usually increased. With acute hemorrhage, the full response of the bone marrow does not appear for about 7–10 days. In the first few days the hematologic picture resembles a hypoproliferative process, with a reticulocyte index of 1 and an E:M ratio of 1:3. Polychromasia is present, but not prominent. Red cell progenitors increase shortly after the blood loss, but it takes time for the red cells to reach sufficient maturity to leave the marrow as young reticulocytes or even as nucleated red cells in the form of polychromatophilic or orthochromatic normoblasts. During this stage the response resembles ineffective erythropoiesis, with a reticulocyte index of 1–2 and an E:M ratio, though increased, still <1:1. Polychromasia is more prominent than earlier. Finally, after 7–10 days the hematologic findings resemble a hemolytic anemia, with a reticulocyte index of >3 and an E:M ratio of 1:1 or greater. Polychromasia is impressive at this stage. Because red cells are not undergoing increased destruction during this recovery period, however, the indirect bilirubin and LDH levels are normal.

These two ways of classifying anemia—by morphology or red cell kinetics—are not mutually exclusive. One useful approach is to use the red cell size in the initial categorization. For macrocytic or microcytic anemias the differential diagnosis is small. For the normochromic, normocytic anemias, however, further analyzing the hematologic information in terms of hypoproliferative versus hemolytic or hemorrhagic is helpful in distinguishing among the many causes.

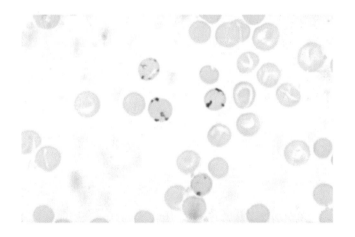

Slide 91: Reticulocyte: New Methylene Blue Stain

Because the erythrocyte's life span is approximately 120 days, about 0.8% of the red cells need to be replaced daily by young cells released from the bone marrow. These immature cells still contain ribosomal RNA that can be precipitated and stained by supravital dyes, such as new methylene blue or brilliant cresyl blue. The blood and stain are mixed together and allowed to sit for about 15 minutes before the films are prepared and air-dried. The cells containing blue granules or reticulum are counted as a percentage of total red cells or as an absolute number per volume (mm³, L, or μL). Automated methods employ a substance, such as thiazole orange, that binds to RNA and fluoresces. In this slide the four erythrocytes demonstrating the finely dispersed, netlike aggregates of precipitated blue RNA are reticulocytes.

MICROCYTIC ANEMIAS

Table 3. Causes of Microcytic Anemia

Iron deficiency
Anemia of chronic disease
Thalassemias
Abnormal hemoglobins (C, E)
Sideroblastic anemias

Iron Deficiency Anemia

The most frequent cause of iron deficiency is chronic blood loss. In pre-menopausal women the source is usually menstruation. In men and in postmenopausal women, the usual cause is gastrointestinal hemorrhage. Less common sources include hemoptysis, epistaxis, hematuria, and intrapulmonary hemorrhage from such disorders as Goodpasture's syndrome or idiopathic hemosiderosis. A rare cause is intravascular hemolysis with iron loss in the urine in the form of ferritin, hemosiderin, and hemoglobin. This process may occur in such disorders as paroxysmal nocturnal hemoglobinuria or red cell fragmentation from a prosthetic cardiac valve.

Iron deficiency anemia occasionally results from inadequate dietary intake. Most foods, including the majority of fruits and vegetables, provide little absorbable iron. Exceptions are meat, fish, poultry, beans, and peas. Since adult males have sparse iron losses, primarily a small amount in the stool, they need little dietary iron, and deficiency from an inadequate intake is rare. When there is increased iron utilization, as in infants or during growth, or when there is concurrent blood loss, particularly in menstruating women, ordinary dietary intake may be inadequate, especially since women and young children often consume less than the recommended minimum daily requirement. An additional contributing factor in women is that during pregnancy iron is diverted to the fetus for hematopoiesis, and after delivery iron is lost through lactation.

Iron absorption can occur anywhere in the intestine, but it is most efficient in the duodenum. Occasionally, iron deficiency results from malabsorption due to disease of the small intestine or following gastric resection, which may contribute to inadequate absorption by causing intestinal contents to travel more rapidly through the duodenum or to bypass it by entering surgically created anastomoses.

Mild iron deficiency anemia is commonly asymptomatic, but the clinical features of severe anemia may emerge as the hematocrit decreases. Two unusual findings are pica—the bizarre craving to ingest certain unusual substances, such as clay, ice, dirt, or cardboard—and spooning of the nails (koilonychia).

In iron deficiency anemia, the serum iron level is decreased, the total iron-binding capacity increased, and the percent saturation diminished to less than 20%. In addition, the serum ferritin level is usually low, but, since the presence of inflammation can elevate it, the concurrence of iron deficiency anemia and an inflammatory process may result in a normal or nearly normal serum ferritin level. An examination of the blood smear and characteristic findings in these serum studies usually allow a confident diagnosis of iron deficiency anemia to be made, but if these are confusing, a definitive diagnosis can be made on iron stains of a bone marrow aspirate or on the basis of a hematologic response to a therapeutic trial of iron replacement.

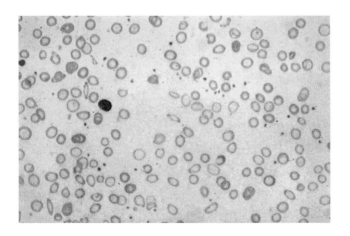

Slide 92. Iron Deficiency Anemia

When iron deficiency anemia is recent and mild, the smear and erythrocyte indices (MCV, MCH, MCHC) may be normal. An early change is anisocytosis, reflected by increased red cell distribution width (RDW) on automated counters. With increased severity—hematocrits typically less than 36 in men, 30 in women—the MCV and MCHC diminish, and the major changes on the smear are anisocytosis, microcytosis, hypochromia, and poikilocytosis, including hypochromic, elongated, elliptical erythrocytes ("pencil cells"). Tiny microcytes and occasional target cells may be present, as may polychromatophilia. Basophilic stippling is rarely found, and Pappenheimer bodies, which contain iron granules, are absent. Some normal-appearing red cells are common. Occasionally, mild leukopenia is present. In many cases thrombocytosis occurs, especially with active bleeding. In this slide, the red cells vary widely in shape and size. Comparison with the lymphocyte reveals that the erythrocytes are microcytic. Their increased central pallor indicates hypochromia. Several long, thin pencil cells and tiny microcytes are present. Thrombocytosis is apparent.

Thalassemias

In normal adults, over 90% of hemoglobin is Hb A, which consists of four polypeptide chains, two α and two β ($\alpha_2\beta_2$). A small fraction is Hb A$_2$, composed of two α-chains and two δ-chains ($\alpha_2\delta_2$). In fetal life the major hemoglobin is Hb F ($\alpha_2\gamma_2$), the production of which decreases shortly before birth as formation of β-chains begins. At birth about 75% of the infant's hemoglobin is Hb F, but by 6 months it decreases to below 5%, and in adult life it constitutes less than 1% of the total hemoglobin. The thalassemias consist of a group of inherited disorders with impaired synthesis of one or more of the globin chains, leading to production of a defective hemoglobin, which causes microcytic hypochromic red cells. In addition, when one type of polypeptide chain is absent or decreased, the other, unaffected chain is not bound and in its free form can damage red cells or their precursors. The thalassemias are labeled according to the chain whose production is impaired: β-thalassemia when β-chains are either absent or decreased, α-thalassemia when the α-chains are affected. These are the two most important types, although other forms exist (e.g., γ-, δ-, and $\delta\beta$-thalassemias).

The β-thalassemias are common in the Mediterranean area, the Middle East, Southeast Asia, China, and parts of India and Pakistan. The clinical consequences of this disorder vary considerably, ranging from severe (thalassemia major) to moderate (thalassemia intermedia) to mild (thalassemia minor), depending on whether the inheritance is homozygous or heterozygous and whether the abnormal gene leads to no β-chain production (β^o) or a decreased amount (β^+).

In homozygous disease, with little or no β-chain production and normal α-chain formation, an excess of α-chains develops. These are unable to combine to form a viable hemoglobin, and consequently precipitate in red cell precursors, destroying many in the bone marrow (ineffective erythropoiesis). Red cells with these inclusions that do reach the circulation have a shortened life span, being prematurely destroyed by macrophages in the liver, spleen, and bone marrow. Because substantial amounts of Hb F are present at birth, affected infants are well until γ-chain synthesis decreases and anemia begins to appear. With sufficient transfusions to maintain relatively normal hemoglobin levels, children grow and develop normally until the iron overload problems of repetitive transfusions emerge. Untreated or inadequately transfused patients have stunted growth. Increased erythropoiesis can produce systemic features of hypermetabolism, such as fever, wasting, and hyperuricemia. In addition, expanded marrow cavities can cause fractures in long bones and can enlarge the diameters of the skull and maxillary region, producing distorted head and facial appearances. Continued phagocytosis of abnormal erythrocytes causes splenomegaly, which can result in secondary thrombocytopenia and leukopenia. In thalassemia major, the anemia is severe, and erythrocytes demonstrate anisocytosis and poikilocytosis, including elliptocytes, teardrop cells, and erythrocytes with other bizarre shapes. Hypochromia is very impressive, and microcytosis is typically apparent, but the pallid cells are flat and spread out on drying, causing them to appear larger than their MCV would suggest. Target cells are common, nucleated red cells are usually numerous, and basophilic stippling is prominent. Red cell inclusions having the same color as hemoglobin and representing excess α-chains may appear on Wright's stain, especially after splenectomy, but are more obvious on methyl violet stains. The bone marrow demonstrates erythroid hyperplasia with basophilic stippling and decreased hemoglobin content of erythroblasts. Red cell inclusions are present in erythroid cells, and iron content is increased.

In thalassemia intermedia the disease is less severe, with a later onset, milder clinical features, and lower transfusion requirements. This disorder usually develops from the inheritance of two β-thalassemia mutations, both mild or one mild and one severe. The blood film resembles that of thalassemia major, but the hematocrit is usually in the 20s.

The heterozygous state for β-thalassemia (thalassemia minor or thalassemia trait) causes no clinical problems, and anemia is mild or absent, but the blood smear is abnormal. The cells are microcytic and hypochromic, with an MCV of about 50–70 and an MCH of 20–22. Target cells, poikilocytosis, and basophilic stippling are typical. The marrow exhibits mild erythroid hyperplasia and rare red cell inclusions. Hemoglobin electrophoresis demonstrates Hb A_2 levels that are about twice normal (5%) and an Hb A_2/Hb A ratio of 1:20, rather than the normal 1:40. Hb F is increased (>2%) in about one-half of patients.

Four gene loci govern α-globin chain production. The four α-thalassemias are α-thalassemia-2, in which one focus fails to function; α-thalassemia-1, with two abnormal genes; Hb H disease, with three; and Hb Bart's, with four. No hematologic abnormalities occur with α-thalassemia-2, a silent, asymptomatic carrier state. With α-thalassemia-1, a benign disorder found primarily in people of Asian, Mediterranean, and African descent, the hematologic findings consist of microcytosis, hypochromia, and slight anisocytosis and poikilocytosis. Anemia is absent or mild.

When three gene foci are defective, α-chain production diminishes markedly, and the excess β-chains form tetramers of Hb H, which, being soluble, does not precipitate in the marrow to damage erythroid precursors and cause ineffective erythropoiesis. Instead, it remains in the mature circulating erythrocytes, but precipitates as they age, with the formation of inclusion bodies. These cells are prematurely destroyed in the spleen, causing hemolytic anemia. This disorder occurs predominantly in Asians, and occasionally in individuals of Mediterranean or African descent. Splenomegaly and osseous changes similar to those in β-thalassemia intermedia may occur; the anemia is usually moderate, with hematocrits of 20–30. The blood smear shows marked hypochromia, microcytosis, basophilic stippling, and polychromasia. Poikilocytosis is typical and may include target cells, teardrop cells, and fragmented erythrocytes, as well as nucleated red cells. Heinz body preparations show multiple small erythrocyte inclusions, which are precipitated Hb H. On hemoglobin electrophoresis, about 3–30% of the total is Hb H.

With four genes defective, α-chains are absent, and γ-chain tetramers, Hb Bart's, form in the fetus. These carry oxygen poorly, causing tissue hypoxia, and are somewhat unstable, leading to hemolysis and anemia. This combination causes heart and liver failure, resulting in massive edema (hydrops fetalis) and intrauterine death. This disorder occurs almost exclusively in Southeast Asians. Its importance in adult hematology is that a history of hydrops fetalis in an Asian family suggests a form of α-thalassemia in the parents.

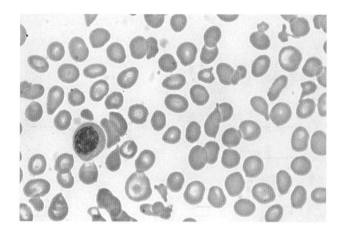

Slide 93. β-Thalassemia Trait

Although people with β-thalassemia trait are hetero-zygous for a condition that causes decreased synthesis of the β-globin chains in hemoglobin, most are not anemic, but their red cells are generally markedly microcytic and hypochromic. The erythrocytes may display mild to substantial poikilocytosis, and target cells are commonly present. Sometimes coarse baso-philic stippling and elliptocytosis are prominent, and occasionally schistocytes and teardrop cells appear. In this slide, target cells are present; other abnormal erythrocytes include elliptocytes, teardrop cells, mi-crocytes, and irregularly shaped cells. The presence of a normal small lymphocyte permits size compar-ison.

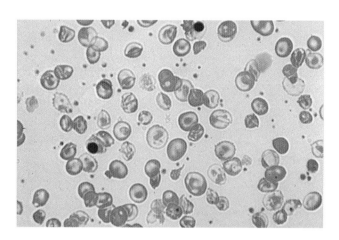

Slide 94. β-Thalassemia Major

With β-thalassemia major, marked microcytosis, hy-pochromia, and anisocytosis occur. Poikilocytosis is prominent, with target cells, elliptocytes, fragments, and teardrop cells. Basophilic stippling and Pappen-heimer bodies are frequent, as are nucleated red cells. This slide shows poikilocytosis, anisocytosis, and marked hypochromia, some cells being astonishingly pale. Two nucleated erythrocytes are visible, and prominent target cells are present. Platelets are in-creased.

MACROCYTIC ANEMIAS

Table 4. Causes of Macrocytic Anemias

Folate deficiency
B_{12} deficiency
Hypothyroidism
Myelodysplasia
Medications that impair DNA synthesis
Hemolysis/hemorrhage causing early bone marrow
  release of young, large cells
Liver disease
Alcoholism (macrocytosis without anemia)

Megaloblastic Anemias

In megaloblastic anemias, impaired DNA synthesis causes defective nuclear maturation of hematopoietic cells in the bone marrow. In erythrocyte precursors, division of nuclei diminishes, while cytoplasmic growth, regulated by RNA, remains unimpeded, resulting in large cells with greater cytoplasm than normal (megaloblasts). As these cells differentiate, the nuclear chromatin condenses more slowly than usual, giving a lacy appearance whose immaturity contrasts with the increasing amount of hemoglobin in the cytoplasm, a feature described as nuclear-cytoplasmic dyssynchrony. In megaloblastic anemias, the cytoplasm is usually more mature than the nucleus, but sometimes a few cells demonstrate the reverse. Granulocyte precursors are also larger than normal, and especially characteristic cells are the giant metamyelocytes and bands, which have a size two to three times normal, a shape that is often unusual, a nucleus with poorly condensed chromatin, and a vacuolated cytoplasm. Megakaryocytes are hypersegmented and have a "megaloblastic" nuclear chromatin. The bone marrow shows hypercellularity, but the common presence of anemia and a decreased reticulocyte count in the peripheral blood indicates that many of the erythrocytes, rather than reaching maturity and entering the systemic circulation, are destroyed in the bone marrow, a condition called ineffective erythropoiesis. This intramedullary hemolysis causes increases in serum iron, unconjugated bilirubin, and LDH levels, which are further elevated by extramedullary hemolysis, since the red cell life span in the circulation is decreased by 30–50%.

Early in the course of disease, the only finding in the peripheral blood may be red cell macrocytosis, usually between 110 and 130 fl, but sometimes higher, especially as anemia develops and worsens. When the red cell count diminishes, other abnormalities emerge, including anisocytosis, poikilocytosis, teardrop cells, schistocytes, basophilic stippling, and sometimes Howell-Jolly bodies. Even in the presence of significant anemia, polychromatophilic cells are absent or sparse, and the reticulocyte count is low. Leukopenia and thrombocytopenia may occur, particularly when anemia is severe. Two findings on a blood smear strongly suggest a megaloblastic process: some of the macrocytes are oval, a feature absent in nonmegaloblastic causes of macrocytosis, and polymorphonuclear leukocytes usually demonstrate hypersegmentation, defined as >5% of neutrophils having five segments or any having six or more. Sometimes circulating megaloblasts and giant platelets are visible.

The most common causes of megaloblastic anemia are deficiencies in vitamin B_{12} (cobalamin) and folate, whose hematologic features are indistinguishable. Some drugs can cause megaloblastic anemias by impairing DNA synthesis, including various cytotoxic agents used in cancer chemotherapy (such as cytosine arabinoside and cyclophosphamide), certain anticonvulsants (such as phenytoin), and medications interfering with folate metabolism (such as methotrexate or trimethoprim). Rare causes are various inborn errors of metabolism.

Cobalamins are molecules with a central cobalt atom that are important in DNA synthesis. Strictly speaking, vitamin B_{12} is cyanocobalamin, a stable product used for therapy but not normally found in the human body. Often the term vitamin B_{12}, however, is loosely employed for all cobalamins. Microbes present in the soil, water, or the intestinal tract of animals synthesize these substances. They are not found in plants unless contaminated by microbes, and the dietary source for humans is thus meat, poultry, seafood, and dairy products. The average diet in Western countries contains 5–30 μg of cobalamin, the recommended daily allowance being 5 μg. The total body content is about 2–5 mg in adults, about 1 mg of which is in the liver. Daily losses are very small, and even with no intake, depletion sufficient to cause cobalamin deficiency takes years. Only strict vegetarians are likely to develop cobalamin deficiency on the basis of inadequate ingestion alone. Instead, cobalamin deficiency in adults almost always develops from impaired absorption. Normally, cobalamin binds with substances in the gastric juice called R proteins. When this complex reaches the duodenum, pancreatic enzymes release the cobalamin, which then binds with intrinsic factor, a glycoprotein produced by the parietal cells of the stomach. Intrinsic factor receptors are present on the mucosa of the ileum, especially in its terminal portion, where cobalamin is normally absorbed.

Diminished cobalamin absorption may occur in the ileum because of ileal resection or disease, such as radiation enteritis, lymphoma, or Crohn's disease. Cobalamin can be removed from the small intestine by a fish tapeworm, *Diphyllobothrium latum,* found primarily in Canada, Alaska, and the Baltic Sea and acquired by eating undercooked fish or fish roe. In small intestinal disorders with markedly impaired motility, such as systemic sclerosis, or with anatomic lesions associated with intestinal stasis, such as diverticula and surgical blind loops, bacteria can proliferate and consume cobalamin. Malabsorption of cobalamin in the small intestine can also occur from pancreatic disease when insufficient pancreatic enzymes are present to release cobalamin from the R protein binding it. The major cause of cobalamin deficiency, however, is an inadequate supply of intrinsic factor, either from surgical resection of gastric parietal cells or, most commonly, from a disease causing chronic inflammation and mucosal atrophy in the fundus and body of the stomach, probably through immune mechanisms.

This disorder, pernicious anemia, occurs predominantly in older adults, with a median age at diagnosis of about 60. About 20% have a familial history of the disease, many are of northern European descent, and some have other autoimmune conditions such as vitiligo, Hashimoto's thyroiditis, and Graves' disease. About 90% of patients have serum antibodies to parietal cells, compared to about 5% in the general population, and approximately 60% have serum antibodies to intrinsic factor, which is rare in healthy people. Histologic examination of gastric specimens demonstrates mucosal atrophy, markedly diminished parietal cells, and an infiltration of the submucosa and lamina propria by lymphocytes and plasma cells. As a result, gastric secretion is reduced, causing achlorhydria and decreased intrinsic factor production. The risk of gastric carcinoma in pernicious anemia is about 2–3 times that of the normal population.

The clinical features of cobalamin deficiency are diverse. Those due to anemia itself include pallor, fatigue, and dyspnea. Nonspecific gastrointestinal complaints are diarrhea, anorexia, and weight loss. Many patients have attacks of glossitis, with soreness and beefy redness, especially of the anterior half of the tongue; when the episode resolves, papillae may be absent, causing a smooth, glazed surface. Cobalamin deficiency causes impaired myelination of nerves, leading to degeneration of white matter in the spinal cord ("subacute combined degeneration") and cerebrum. Involvement of the dorsal column of the spinal cord causes loss of vibratory sensation and proprioception, with patients complaining of numbness and tingling, initially in the feet but later in the hands as well (stocking-glove distribution). Diminished proprioception can cause difficulty with gait and a positive Romberg's sign. Lateral column damage leads to limb weakness, spasticity, hyperactive reflexes, and a positive Babinski's sign. Depression and impaired memory are the most common cerebral manifestations, but confusion, delusions, and hallucinations can also occur.

Serum cobalamin levels are low in most patients with pernicious anemia, but false positives and negatives occasionally occur. In those circumstances, other studies may help. One cobalamin-dependent enzyme, methylmalonyl CoA mutase, participates in the disposal of propionate generated during the breakdown of valine and isoleucine. When inadequate cobalamin leads to diminished amounts of this enzyme, methylmalonic acid accumulates, and measurements of its serum level or urinary excretion are highly accurate in diagnosing cobalamin deficiency. A useful approach for the occasional patient with confusing findings is a therapeutic trial of parenteral cobalamin. A brisk reticulocytosis occurs 5–7 days later if cobalamin deficiency is present.

A Schilling test can determine the pathogenesis of cobalamin deficiency. In healthy people, orally administered radiolabeled cobalamin is absorbed from the gastrointestinal tract and later excreted in the urine. In patients with pernicious anemia, the cobalamin is not absorbed normally, and therefore its urinary excretion is decreased. When ingested with concurrent oral intrinsic factor, however, the cobalamin is absorbed and excreted normally. With other forms of intestinal malabsorption, urinary excretion remains low despite intrinsic factor. When bacterial overgrowth is the cause, the Schilling test may become normal after a course of antibiotic therapy active against intestinal bacteria.

Unlike cobalamin, folate is not present in high quantities in the body. Its store is estimated to be about 5–10 mg. Since the normal daily requirement is 50–100 μg, only a few weeks to months of decreased intake is necessary before deficiency develops and hematologic abnormalities emerge. The richest food sources are vegetables, liver, and fruit. Inadequate dietary ingestion, a common cause of folate deficiency, may occur because of poverty, ignorance, food fads, and alcoholism. With excessive ethanol, further mechanisms lead to folate deficiency: alcohol itself can increase urinary folate excretion, impede its storage in the liver, and diminish folate absorption, which occurs primarily in the duodenum and jejunum. Malabsorption of folate may also develop in extensive disorders of the small bowel, such as sprue, Crohn's disease, lymphoma, amyloidosis, Whipple's disease, and substantial intestinal resection. Deficiency is frequent when requirements for folate increase, as in pregnancy and conditions causing accelerated cell turnover, such as leukemia, acute exacerbations of chronic hemolytic anemia, multiple myeloma, and exfoliative dermatitis. Some medications, including anticonvulsants and sulfasalazine, can cause folate deficiency by altering its metabolism.

The symptoms of folate deficiency relate primarily to anemia. In contrast to cobalamin deficiency it rarely, if ever, causes neurologic damage. The most useful diagnostic test is determination of the serum folate level, which reflects folate intake. When folate ingestion first diminishes, however, the serum level will decrease before tissue stores are depleted, and when folate ingestion increases, the serum level will rise before tissue stores are replaced. The red cell folate level, which remains relatively constant during the erythrocyte's life span, is a better indicator of tissue folate status, but it is often normal when the folate deficiency is acute. Moreover, it is decreased in many patients with cobalamin deficiency and so cannot be used to accurately distinguish between these two causes of megaloblastic anemia. Usually, concurrent serum levels of cobalamin and folate will allow a reliable discrimination. Occasionally, however, both will be decreased. The possible causes of this situation include (1) simultaneous deficiencies in both substances, a very unusual event; (2) cobalamin deficiency with a recent decrease in folate intake but still adequate tissue stores; and (3) cobalamin deficiency with an unexplained decrease in serum folate levels, which occurs in some patients with cobalamin deficiency and apparently normal folate intake. These possibilities can usually be sorted out by measuring serum or urine methylmalonic acid or by a therapeutic trial monitoring a reticulocyte response following replacement with *physiologic* doses of either cobalamin (100 μg daily) or folate (100–200 μg) given parenterally. Higher doses are misleading, since the hematologic findings of cobalamin deficiency correct with large amounts of folate and those of folate deficiency improve with higher doses of cobalamin. Misdiagnosis of cobalamin deficiency because of a hematologic improvement with folate therapy is a very serious error, since the neurologic abnormalities are unaffected and will progress without cobalamin replacement.

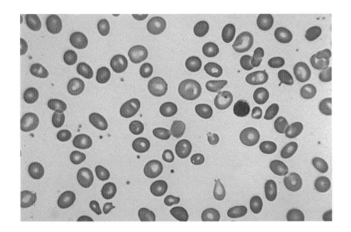

Slide 95. Folate or Vitamin B₁₂ Deficiency

These two deficiencies demonstrate identical appearances on the blood smear. The characteristic red cells are macrocytic, some of these are oval (macroovalocytes), and central pallor may be absent. Anisocytosis is always present, not all cells being macrocytic; rather, a spectrum of size occurs, ranging from very large to microcytic. Poikilocytosis is prominent as well, with teardrops and fragments (schistocytes) common, especially with severe anemia. Basophilic stippling can occur, and nucleated red cells with large nuclei (megaloblasts) may be present. Neutrophilic hypersegmentation and macropolycytes (large hypersegmented neutrophils) are typically prominent. In this slide, a comparison of the erythrocytes with the lymphocyte reveals that many of the red cells are larger than normal, and some are oval. Anisocytosis and poikilocytosis are apparent, and two microcytic cells are located close to the lymphocyte.

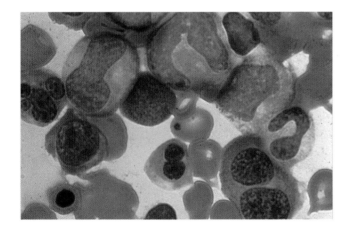

Slide 96. Folate or Vitamin B₁₂ Deficiency: Bone Marrow Aspirate

The bone marrow in these two deficiencies shows hyperplasia and the characteristic pattern of megaloblastic anemia (see slide 61). The erythroid cell situated in the lower central area of this slide exhibits both dysplastic (irregular nucleus contours giving the nucleus a "pinched" appearance) and megaloblastic (fully matured cytoplasm with pink hemoglobin but still retaining a nucleus—the so-called "nuclear-cytoplasmic maturation dyssynchrony") features. The binucleated erythroid precursor in the right lower corner, however, has a somewhat mature-appearing nucleus with clumped, closed chromatin, but the cytoplasm displays immature basophilic staining. This feature demonstrates that in some cells in megaloblastic anemias, the nucleus matures more rapidly than the cytoplasm. The three large upper white cells are all giant granulocytes (two metamyelocytes and a central band), and an erythrocyte in the center contains a Howell-Jolly body, sometimes present in megaloblastic anemias.

HEMOLYTIC ANEMIAS

In hemolytic anemias the erythrocytes' life span in the peripheral blood, normally about 120 days, substantially shortens because of red cell destruction. Hemolytic anemias are generally categorized by two systems—the site of hemolysis or the location of the abnormality responsible for the hemolysis, characterized as being either intrinsic or extrinsic to the red cell.

The site of hemolysis may be intravascular, in which case the erythrocyte is destroyed in the circulation, or extravascular, in which case the red cell destruction occurs within macrophages in the spleen, liver, or bone marrow. Intravascular hemolysis is typically severe and results from (1) mechanical damage to the red cell due to prosthetic valves, the presence of fibrin within the vasculature (microangiopathic hemolytic anemia), or thermal injury to the erythrocytes from serious burns; (2) infections or toxins, such as *Clostridium perfringens* bacteremia, severe *falciparum* malaria, or certain snake venoms; or (3) complement-mediated damage to red cells, as with paroxysmal nocturnal hemoglobinuria, ABO-incompatible blood transfusions, and cold agglutinins. Intravascular hemolysis liberates hemoglobin into the bloodstream, where it binds to haptoglobin, this complex being removed by the liver. A reduced serum haptoglobin level, therefore, is one finding in intravascular hemolysis, but it also occurs in extravascular hemolysis. When the amount of free hemoglobin in the circulation exceeds the binding capacity of haptoglobin, it makes the plasma pink and is filtered through the kidneys. The urine may become red and the dipstick testing for blood turns positive in the absence of erythrocytes on urine microscopy. The renal tubular cells, which reabsorb some of the hemoglobin and convert it to hemosiderin, are shed into the urine. Iron stains of urinary sediment demonstrate the hemosiderin within these renal tubular cells and confirm ongoing or recent intravascular hemolysis, even when hemoglobin is undetectable in the plasma or urine.

In the remaining hemolytic anemias, accounting for most cases, red cell destruction is extravascular. The causes are (1) an abnormal environment in the circulation produced by infections, drugs, or immunologic processes; (2) red cell membrane defects, such as hereditary spherocytosis; (3) erythrocyte metabolic defects, such as deficiencies in pyruvate kinase or G6PD; and (4) hemoglobin structural defects, such as sickle cell anemia or hemoglobin C.

The other classification of hemolytic anemias distinguishes between disorders intrinsic to the red cell, generally hereditary, and those extrinsic to the red cell, generally acquired. The intrinsic disorders include (1) abnormal hemoglobins, such as HbS or HbC; (2) enzyme defects, such as deficiencies in G6PD; and (3) membrane abnormalities, such as hereditary spherocytosis or elliptocytosis. The extrinsic abnormalities are (1) immunologic—*alloantibodies*, such as those associated with ABO incompatibility; *autoantibodies*, as in warm (IgG) or cold (IgM) antibody hemolytic anemias; or *drug-induced antibodies*; (2) mechanical factors, such as trauma from prosthetic valves or fibrin deposition in small vessels in microangiopathic hemolytic anemias; (3) infections and toxins, such as *falciparum* malaria or certain snake venoms; and (4) severe hypophosphatemia.

In hemolytic anemias the reticulocyte index is >3 and the absolute reticulocyte count is >100,000/mm^3. The MCV may be normal or increased, depending on how many large, immature erythrocytes have prematurely left the bone marrow in response to the anemia. The indirect bilirubin is elevated and accounts for >80% of the total bilirubin. The serum LDH level is increased, and the serum haptoglobin is commonly diminished. A blood smear may be very helpful in demonstrating (1) polychromatophilia, confirming the early departure of red cells from the bone marrow; (2) abnormalities in red cell shape, such as fragments, sickle cells, spherocytes, or bite cells, which may be diagnostic or at least highly suggestive of the cause; (3) red cell agglutination, indicating IgM-mediated disease; (4) organisms, such as *Plasmodium falciparum* or *Babesia*; and (5) erythrophagocytosis, seen especially with red cell damage from immune mechanisms, but also with certain infection or toxins.

Tests useful in suspected intravascular hemolysis include evaluation of the plasma and urine for hemoglobin and an iron stain of the urine sediment to detect hemosiderin. For immune-related hemolytic anemia, Coombs' tests to demonstrate IgG and complement on the red cell or in the serum and cold-agglutinin tests looking for IgM are indicated. With suspected hemoglobinopathies, a hemoglobin electrophoresis is appropriate. Other laboratory evaluations depend on the likely abnormality and may include searching for rare enzyme defects.

Table 5. Causes of Hemolysis (by Site of Abnormality)

Intrinsic to the red cell	Extrinsic to the red cell
Abnormal hemoglobins	Immunologic
Sickle cell anemia	Warm antibody
Hemoglobin C, E, etc.	Cold antibody
Enzyme defects	Drugs
Glucose-6-phosphate dehydrogenase deficiency	Mechanical
Pyruvate kinase deficiency, etc.	March hemoglobinuria
Membrane abnormalities	Traumatic cardiac hemolytic anemia
Hereditary spherocytosis, elliptocytosis	Microangiopathic hemolytic anemia
Acanthocytosis	Infectious
Paroxysmal nocturnal hemoglobinuria	Malaria
	Clostridium perfringens infection
	Chemicals
	Hypersplenism

Table 6. Causes of Hemolysis (by Site of Destruction)

Intravascular hemolysis
  Mechanical
    March hemoglobinuria
    Cardiac hemolytic anemia
    Vasculitis
  Osmotic
    Distilled water
  Chemical or thermal damage
    Alpha toxin of *Clostridium perfringens*
    Burns
    Snake venoms
    Drugs in patients with G6PD deficiency
  Complement damage
    Cold agglutinins
    Paroxysmal nocturnal hemoglobinuria
    Isoantibody plus complement

Extravascular hemolysis
  Environmental disorders
    Infections
    Drug-induced
    Immune-mediated
    Hemolytic-uremic syndrome
  Membrane defects
    Hereditary spherocytosis
    Hereditary elliptocytosis
    Acanthocytosis
    Paroxysmal nocturnal hemoglobinuria
  Metabolic defects
    Phosphogluconate pathway (e.g., G6PD deficiency)
    Embden-Meyerhof pathway (e.g., pyruvate kinase deficiency)
  Abnormal hemoglobins
    Hemoglobinopathies
    Unstable hemoglobins

Sickle Cell Anemia

Sickle cell anemia occurs with the inheritance of a β^s gene from each parent. This gene, which encodes the β-globin subunit of hemoglobin, is most prevalent in the populations of tropical Africa, especially in the eastern part, but it also occurs in people from Mediterranean countries, Saudi Arabia, and portions of India. In the United States, it is present in about 8% of blacks and, accordingly, sickle cell anemia (the homozygous state) occurs in about 1 of 625 black infants.

Because of a single substitution of thymine for adenine in this gene, the hemoglobin produced differs from hemoglobin A in having valine, rather than glutamic acid, present in the sixth position from the N terminal of the β-chain. When deoxygenated, this abnormal hemoglobin aggregates into large fibers (polymers) that make the red cell rigid and can change its shape into the classic sickle cell. In addition, damage to the erythrocyte membrane occurs, producing dehydrated, shrunken cells that may permanently sickle. These factors lead to chronic hemolysis. When the deoxygenated abnormal cells adhere to the vascular endothelium, they can obstruct the circulation, leading to ischemia or necrosis of areas that these vessels supply. Such vascular occlusion accounts for most of the clinical features of this disease.

One manifestation is painful crises, which commonly last 4–5 days and may involve any tissue but especially the skeleton, abdomen, and chest. Involvement of vessels to the bones causes a gnawing, progressive discomfort, especially in the humerus, tibia, and femur, but also the ribs, causing thoracic pain. Sometimes vascular occlusion causes marrow necrosis and the release of fat particles (emboli) that travel to the lung or other areas. Abdominal crises probably arise from infarcts to the mesentery and abdominal organs, including the spleen.

Some acute events can cause sudden worsening of anemia. In aplastic crises fever occurs and red cell production markedly diminishes, resulting in a rapid decrease in circulating erythrocytes as the chronic hemolysis continues. The most common cause is infection with parvovirus B19, which directly damages the erythroid precursors. Patients typically recover in 5–10 days. A megaloblastic crisis can also develop, in which folate deficiency from inadequate nutrition or concurrent alcoholism decreases erythropoiesis.

Early in life, the dorsa of the hands and feet can swell (dactylitis), often accompanied by fever and leukocytosis; the mechanism is probably avascular necrosis of the bones. Young children may also experience episodes of acute splenic sequestration, in which red cells abruptly accumulate in the spleen, causing pain, splenic enlargement, and increased anemia. As patients age, the spleen becomes shrunken, scarred, and nonfunctional because of repeated infarcts, and sequestration no longer occurs.

Another sudden event is the acute chest syndrome, characterized by fever, dyspnea, chest pain, leukocytosis, and pulmonary infiltrates. Several entities can cause this condition, including infections, pulmonary vascular occlusion, and fat emboli. In some cases the chest pain arises from rib infarcts.

Strokes may also occur, especially in children, and they tend to recur. The predominant cause is occlusion of the major cerebral vessels, but sometimes they arise from subarachnoid or intracerebral hemorrhage.

Priapism can develop in both prepubertal and postpubertal males. Episodes are usually short-lived but often recurrent, and occur from stagnation of blood in the corpora cavernosa. Repeated episodes may lead to fibrosis and impotence.

With repetitive episodes or chronic ischemia, permanent tissue damage can eventuate in many other locations. Avascular necrosis of the femoral head causes persistent pain and abnormal gait, and involvement of the humeral head typically produces protracted shoulder discomfort. Ischemic or necrotic bone predisposes to osteomyelitis, especially from *Salmonella* species. Damage to the kidneys can produce an inability to concentrate the urine normally (hyposthenuria) and impair excretion of hydrogen ion (renal tubular acidosis). Hematuria may occur, sometimes associated with renal papillary necrosis, which also predisposes to urinary infections. Sloughing of the papillae can lead to urinary tract obstruction. Eye complications include proliferative retinopathy because of chronic ischemia, a cause of visual loss and vitreous hemorrhage. The abnormal vessels may bleed into the anterior chamber (hyphema). Persistent or recurrent painful ulcers sometimes form over the distal leg, especially above the malleoli, usually in adulthood. They are more common in males than in females and typically have a deep base with raised margins. Another common finding in older patients is bilirubin gallstones, a complication of chronic hemolysis.

Sickle cell anemia predisposes to infections, not only because of the presence of ischemic or necrotic tissues but also because of decreased splenic function, which impairs antibody production and splenic phagocytosis of organisms. The alternate complement pathway may also be faulty. In childhood the most common serious infections are from *Streptococcus pneumoniae*.

The anemia is normochromic, normocytic, with a hematocrit typically about 15–33. Mild leukocytosis (12–15,000), with increased neutrophils, and thrombocytosis (about 450,000) are common. The reticulocyte count is usually 10–20%.

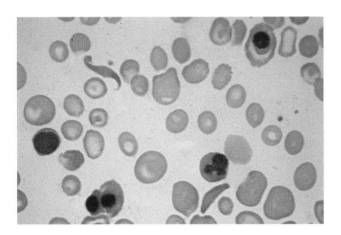

Slide 97. Sickle Cell Anemia

The blood film characteristically demonstrates the crescent-shaped sickle cells, target cells, polychromasia, basophilic stippling, macrocytosis (from large immature erythrocytes released from the bone marrow in response to the anemia), and nucleated red cells. Except in very young children, Howell-Jolly and Pappenheimer bodies, indicating splenic hypofunction from recurrent infarctions and splenic fibrosis, are usually seen. Often visible are "boat-shaped cells," noncrescentic erythrocytes with points at both ends. In this slide, two sickle cells are present. Comparison of the red cells with the small lymphocyte indicates that many erythrocytes are enlarged, and some of these lack central pallor. The presence of macrocytes, polychromasia in several erythrocytes, and the nucleated red cells indicate early release of erythrocytes from the bone marrow secondary to a severe anemia. Two target cells lie below one of the sickle cells.

Hemoglobin C Disease

Hemoglobin C occurs commonly in West Africans and in about 2–3% of African Americans. Patients may be homozygous (CC), heterozygous with normal hemoglobin A (hemoglobin C trait), heterozygous with sickle cells (SC disease), or heterozygous with β-thalassemia. Red cells containing hemoglobin C are abnormally rigid, and their fragmentation may lead to microspherocytes. Their life span is shortened to about 30–35 days.

With hemoglobin C trait, anemia is absent. Blood smears show increased target cells and sometimes hypochromic, microcytic erythrocytes. Electrophoresis typically demonstrates that 30–40% of the hemoglobin is C and 50–60% is A.

In homozygous (CC) disease, splenomegaly is usually present. Both aplastic crises and cholelithiasis may occur. Mild to moderate hemolytic anemia is present, with hematocrits in the mid-20s to 30s and reticulocyte counts typically 2–6%. The erythrocytes may be microcytic and are usually more dense than usual, as reflected in an increased MCHC. Target cells are abundant, and numerous small, dense, and irregularly shaped red cells are present. Crystals of oxygenated hemoglobin C are sometimes visible on peripheral smears as brick-shaped objects, usually within an erythrocyte otherwise devoid of hemoglobin. Polychromatophilia and nucleated red cells, consistent with hemolysis, may be apparent. On electrophoresis, hemoglobin C predominates, A is absent, and F is slightly increased.

With hemoglobin C/β-thalassemia, mild to moderate hemolytic anemia is typical. The blood smear shows microcytosis, hypochromia, target cells, and the small, irregular erythrocytes described above. Hemoglobin C crystals may be visible as well. Electrophoresis typically demonstrates 65–80% Hb C, 20–30% Hb A, and 2–5% Hb F.

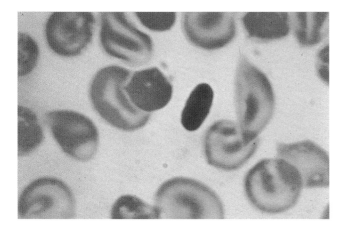

Slide 98. Hemoglobin C Disease

In this specimen from a patient with hemoglobin C disease (homozygous for Hb C), the smear shows numerous target cells and one erythrocyte containing a Hb C crystal, a densely red, blocklike rod.

Hemoglobin SC Disease

Although the red cells in SC disease sickle, causing vascular occlusion, this disorder is milder than sickle cell disease, and life expectancy is nearly normal. It occurs in about 1 in 800 black infants in the United States. Growth and development are usually unaffected. Acute painful episodes (crises) are less frequent and typically shorter than in sickle cell disease. Aseptic necrosis of the humeral and femoral heads, however, may occur. The spleen is usually enlarged and, although susceptible to infarcts, does not become obliterated as in sickle cell disease. Patients with SC disease may suddenly develop the acute splenic sequestration syndrome, especially when at high altitudes: red cells rapidly accumulate in the spleen, causing abdominal pain, progressive splenic enlargement with tenderness, and abrupt decreases in hematocrit, sometimes producing shock.

Patients have a mildly enhanced susceptibility to infections, primarily with *Streptococcus pneumoniae* and *Hemophilus influenzae.* Spontaneous abortions are increased, but the leg ulcerations and neurologic complications seen in sickle cell disease are uncommon. Proliferative retinopathy, however, is more frequent in SC than SS disease.

The hematocrit typically exceeds 27, and the red cells are usually normocytic, but denser than normal, with an increased MCHC characteristic of erythrocytes containing Hb C. Target cells are numerous. "Billiard ball" cells, in which a round mass of hemoglobin appears in the erythrocyte with a clear space separating the mass from the red cell membrane, are a characteristic finding. The erythrocytes are often dense and disfigured, sometimes with branching projections, and they may contain clusters of Hb C crystals of various sizes and shapes, which create straight edges and blunt angles. Scanning electron microscopy demonstrates that these red cells have folds in them. Sickle cells, boat-shaped cells, and nucleated red cells are other findings. Polychromasia may be present, and in those with functional asplenia, Howell-Jolly bodies are visible. Hemoglobin electrophoresis reveals about equal amounts of Hb C and Hb S.

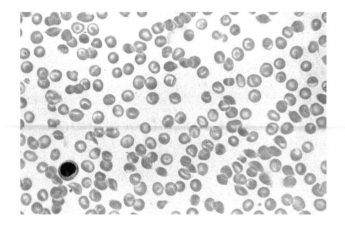

Slide 99. Hemoglobin SC Disease

This slide from a patient with SC disease discloses numerous target cells, a few misshapen cells, and moderate poikilocytosis. The nucleus of the small lymphocyte in the corner allows comparison of the erythrocytes' size.

Red Cell Fragmentation Syndromes

Shear forces within the cardiovascular system can slice off portions of the circulating red cells. The erythrocytes then re-seal their membranes to form fragmented cells (schistocytes). They may appear as triangles, helmet cells, microspherocytes, crescents, or other irregularly shaped erythrocytes that phagocytes remove prematurely from the circulation. The amount of red cell destruction may be sufficient to cause intravascular hemolysis, with hemoglobinemia, hemoglobinuria, and the presence of hemosiderin in the urine. The erythrocyte damage can occur in the heart and great vessels or in the microcirculation.

The most common cardiac etiology is the presence of a prosthetic valve, usually a mechanical device in the aortic position, often associated with regurgitation. Sometimes, however, the prosthetic valve is in the mitral position or is a tissue type. Occasionally, the abnormality is severe aortic stenosis of a native valve, coarctation of the aorta, or an intracardiac patch made from artificial material used to correct anomalies such as septal defects. In each of these situations, excessive turbulence damages the erythrocytes. With chronic mild hemolysis, anemia is absent or slight, the red cells are normal or show some macrocytosis from the presence of immature cells, polychromatophilia is present, and the reticulocyte count is elevated. With more severe hemolysis, erythrocyte fragments (schistocytes) appear on the blood smear, the anemia is moderate to profound, the serum bilirubin and LDH levels rise, haptoglobin decreases, and hemosiderin appears in the urine. With protracted intravascular hemolysis, urinary hemoglobin loss may cause iron deficiency, with hypochromic, microcytic red cells.

When diseases affecting the small vessels produce fragmented red cells, the term used is *microangiopathic hemolytic anemia.* In these disorders, endothelial damage or fibrin deposition in the small vessels damages the red cells as they traverse the abnormal vasculature. One cause is disseminated cancer, usually a mucin-producing neoplasm, especially gastric carcinoma, which accounts for about 50% of cases. Most of the other malignancies producing microangiopathic hemolytic anemia originate from the breast, lung, and pancreas. About one-third of patients have leukoerythroblastosis on the blood smear, about one-half have laboratory evidence of disseminated intravascular coagulation, and about 60% have tumor cells detectable on bone marrow specimens.

Some medications can cause microangiopathic hemolytic anemia, such as mitomycin C, ticlopidine, and tamoxifen. The disease usually begins several weeks to months after initiation of the drug, renal failure and thrombocytopenia are common, and laboratory evidence of disseminated intravascular coagulation is absent. A similar syndrome may occur after solid organ or bone marrow transplantation, possibly precipitated by the preceding cytotoxic medications and total body irradiation used for preparation of the transplant.

Other common causes of microangiopathic hemolytic anemia are thrombotic thrombocytopenic purpura, hemolytic-uremic syndrome, malignant hypertension, disseminated intravascular coagulation, and severe hypertension during pregnancy (preeclampsia or eclampsia). Immunologic damage to the vessels that occurs in such disorders as systemic lupus erythematosus, Wegener's granulomatosis, systemic sclerosis, and microscopic polyangiitis can cause microangiopathic hemolytic anemia. It also may arise from the abnormal vasculature of a giant hemangioma (Kasabach-Merritt syndrome) or a hepatic hemangioendothelioma.

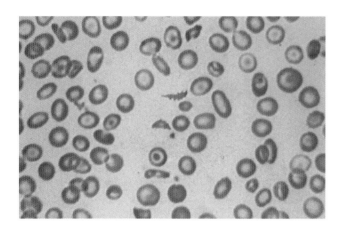

Slide 100. Microangiopathic Hemolytic Anemia

The common findings in microangiopathic hemolytic anemia are numerous fragments, moderate anisocytosis, and poikilocytosis. This slide, from a patient with thrombotic thrombocytopenic purpura, shows marked poikilocytosis with schistocytes, red cell fragments, and other irregularly shaped erythrocytes. Platelets are markedly diminished.

Warm-Antibody Acquired Autoimmune Hemolytic Anemia

In patients with this disorder, the red cell life span decreases because autoantibodies, usually IgG, are optimally active against erythrocytes at body temperature (37°C). These warm antibodies account for about 80–90% of acquired autoimmune hemolytic anemia, the remainder being due to those maximally active at lower temperatures (cold-reactive autoantibodies). In about one-half of cases, an underlying disorder is present, most commonly a lymphoproliferative disease, especially chronic lymphocytic leukemia and lymphomas, but also systemic lupus erythematosus, other inflammatory conditions, some infections, and nonlymphoid malignancies. Certain drugs, such as L-dopa and procainamide, may also cause an autoimmune hemolytic anemia.

In this disorder, IgG, especially IgG1, coats many red cells with or without complement. Macrophages in the spleen and Kupffer cells in the liver trap these erythrocytes, sometimes ingesting them whole. More commonly, they remove a portion of the membrane, and the surviving red cell re-forms as a spherical, rather than biconcave, cell with a smaller diameter. These spherocytes are prominent on a peripheral blood smear, which also discloses evidence of polychromatophilia, indicating the release of immature red cells from the marrow. Erythrocyte fragments, nucleated red cells, and hemophagocytosis by monocytes may also be visible. In addition to anemia, the automated blood count often reveals an increased MCHC, reflecting the presence of the spherocytes. The reticulocyte count is usually increased, as are the serum indirect bilirubin and LDH levels. Immature white cells occasionally appear on the peripheral smear. A bone marrow sample, although usually unnecessary for the diagnosis, shows erythroid hyperplasia. In Evans' syndrome immune thrombocytopenia is also present.

The direct antiglobulin (Coombs') test detects the presence of antibodies and complement on erythrocytes by using a reagent that contains antibodies directed against human immunoglobulin and complement components (primarily C3). This test is nearly always positive in this disorder, but when IgG is present in very small quantities, other diagnostic techniques may be necessary. Autoantibodies unattached to erythrocytes may be present in the serum and are detectable by incubating the patients' serum or plasma with normal red cells, to which the antibodies then attach. These erythrocytes are then tested for the presence of autoantibodies with the Coombs' reagent. This is the indirect antiglobulin or Coombs' test.

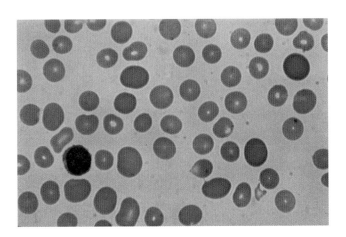

Slide 101. Warm-Antibody Hemolytic Anemia

This slide demonstrates several spherocytes, which have diminished or absent central pallor and are smaller than the nucleus of the small lymphocyte. Several large, polychromatophilic red cells lacking central pallor are present, indicating release of immature erythrocytes in response to the anemia.

Cold-Agglutinin Disease

Cold agglutinins are IgM antierythrocyte antibodies that bind red cells at cold temperatures. They may be polyclonal or monoclonal. Nearly all healthy people have low titers of clinically insignificant polyclonal cold agglutinins. In certain infections, transient, high titers of polyclonal cold agglutinins appear, sometimes causing the abrupt onset of an anemia that is short-lived, but occasionally severe. Infectious mononucleosis and infections with *Mycoplasma pneumoniae* are the two most common causes; the target of the antibodies in the former is typically the i antigen found on the red cell membrane of fetal erythrocytes, while that in the latter is the I antigen found on adult erythrocytes.

The chronic form of cold agglutinin disease, in which a monoclonal antibody appears, typically occurs in older adults, and many have an underlying B-cell neoplasm, such as Waldenström's macroglobulinemia, chronic lymphocytic leukemia, or non-Hodgkin's lymphoma. Exposure to cold may precipitate attacks of acrocyanosis created by agglutination of erythrocytes in cool peripheral areas such as the fingers, toes, nose, and earlobes. It may also cause worsening anemia as the temperature-dependent IgM antibody activates the complement pathway on the red cell membrane, producing intravascular hemolysis, sometimes with sufficient hemoglobinuria to cause acute renal failure. Ordinarily, however, the anemia is mild and stable because the antibody binds to erythrocytes only at temperatures below 37°C; because hepatic macrophages do not avidly phagocytize red cells coated with Cb3, the usual complement component on the membrane; and because the serum Cb3 inactivator system degrades Cb3 into components even less tempting to the macrophages.

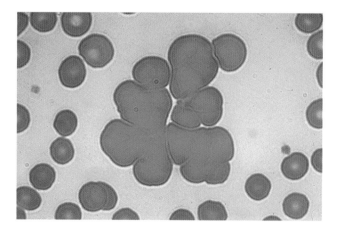

Slide 102. Cold-Agglutinin Hemolytic Anemia

In cold-agglutinin hemolytic anemia the findings on peripheral smear include polychromatophilia, spherocytosis, and, sometimes, erythrocyte agglutination. This slide reveals agglutinated red cells in the center and several spherocytes in the periphery.

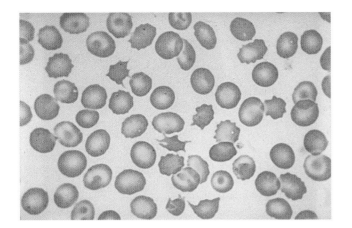

Slide 103. Spur-Cell Anemia

Some patients with severe liver disease, usually alcoholic cirrhosis, develop a hemolytic anemia associated with numerous acanthocytes (spur cells) in the peripheral blood. These form from changes in the cholesterol to phospholipid ratio in the erythrocyte membrane and subsequent alterations produced by passage through the spleen, which destroys many of the cells. The anemia may be profound. This slide, from a patient with severe alcoholic liver disease, shows several acanthocytes and target cells. Platelets are also reduced, probably secondary to alcohol or hypersplenism from portal hypertension.

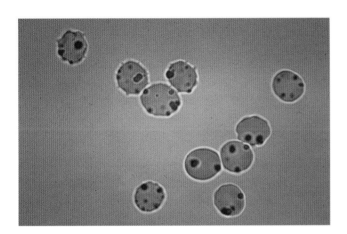

Slide 104. Heinz-Body Anemia: Heinz-Body Preparation

Heinz bodies are fragments of denatured hemoglobin that usually bind to the red cell membrane. They most often occur from oxidative destruction of hemoglobin caused by a medication, especially in patients with G6PD deficiency. These particles are not visible on Wright's stain but are detectable after mixing the erythrocytes with certain basic dyes, such as crystal violet, before making the smear. This slide demonstrates the large, dark-staining inclusions, usually at the cell margins, that are typical of Heinz bodies. Some patients with drug-induced Heinz-body hemolytic anemia but without G6PD deficiency have characteristic red cell abnormalities present on the Wright stain of the peripheral blood, including bite cells (see slide 11) and "blister cells," which have membrane-bound vesicles at the erythrocyte margin.

HYPOPROLIFERATIVE ANEMIAS

Table 7. Causes of Hypoproliferative Anemia

Early iron deficiency
Anemia of chronic disease
Renal disease
Endocrine disorders
  Adrenal insufficiency
  Hypothyroidism
  Hyperthyroidism
  Decreased testosterone
  Panhypopituitarism
Bone marrow disease
  Red cell aplasia
  Aplastic anemia
  Myelodysplasia
  Bone marrow infiltration by malignancy, fibrosis,
    or granulomas
  Myeloproliferative syndromes

Anemia of Chronic Disease

In certain disorders that persist for longer than 1–2 months, especially those with inflammation, infection, and neoplasia, an anemia may develop in which the serum iron and iron-binding capacity are low and the transferrin saturation is diminished, yet the bone marrow iron stores are adequate. Insufficient iron supply to the developing red cells may be a factor in the pathogenesis of the anemia, as may a mildly shortened life span, but the major element apparently is the reduced erythropoietin production and diminished proliferation of erythroid progenitor cells caused by inflammatory cytokines. In about 25% of patients with this anemia, the only chronic disease present is not obviously inflammatory, infectious, or neoplastic but is a disorder such as diabetes mellitus, congestive heart failure, chronic obstructive lung disease, or cardiac ischemia.

Usually the anemia is mild to moderate, with the hematocrit >25, but in about 20% of patients it is lower, and in general, the degree of anemia corresponds with the severity of the underlying disorder. Typically the red cells are normochromic, normocytic. In about 20–30%, however, they are hypochromic (MCHC 26–32) and microcytic. The MCV is rarely <70 fl, and sometimes the erythrocytes demonstrate hypochromia without microcytosis. Overall, hypochromia is present in 40–70% of patients. The smear may disclose mild poikilocytosis and anisocytosis, but these features are less impressive than in iron deficiency, and markedly small and thin cells are absent. Reticulocytes are normal or reduced in number. While the serum iron level is low, as in iron deficiency, the iron-binding capacity is also diminished, whereas it is usually elevated in iron deficiency. The transferrin saturation may be decreased, even to values less than 10%. The most useful serum test is the ferritin level, which is diminished in iron deficiency but increased in the anemia of chronic disease. In mixed-etiology anemia, overlap of these two types of anemias often occurs, however, because inflammatory diseases raise the ferritin level. A value of <30 μg/L in a patient with a chronic disease certainly indicates iron deficiency, and one >100 excludes it, but levels in between are inconclusive. Definitive information in those circumstances can come only from bone marrow samples stained for iron.

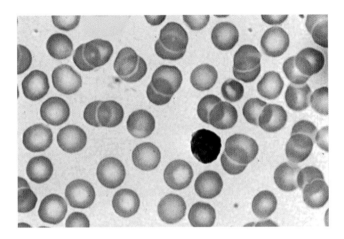

Slide 105. Anemia of Chronic Disease

This smear shows mild microcytosis with normochromic erythrocytes and slight anisocytosis.

Pure Red Cell Aplasia

Pure red cell aplasia is a normochromic, normocytic anemia with a very low reticulocyte count ($<1\%$) and a bone marrow demonstrating normal myeloid cells and megakaryocytes, but a dearth of erythroblasts. It can occur as a congenital disorder (Blackfan-Diamond syndrome) or as an acquired disease that is primary or secondary to medications, neoplasms, immunologic disorders, or infections. In primary acquired pure red cell aplasia the process may arise from an IgG antibody that inhibits erythropoiesis, and the mechanism in some of the secondary causes is also immunologic. With drugs, the process may occur either shortly after initiation of treatment or considerably later, and it typically resolves quickly after discontinuing the medication. The most commonly incriminated agents have been phenytoin, azathioprine, chlorpropamide, and isoniazid, but many others are occasionally responsible. The neoplasms most frequently associated with pure red cell aplasia are thymomas and chronic lymphocytic leukemia, in both of which the frequency is about 5–10%. A few cases have occurred with carcinomas, including those of the lung, kidney, stomach, and breast. The infectious causes are primarily viral, especially with parvovirus B19, infectious mononucleosis, and viral hepatitis; usually the anemia abates when the acute infection resolves. Because red cells normally survive for about 120 days, infection-induced aplasia, typically short-lived, is usually clinically inapparent except in chronic hemolytic anemias, such as hereditary spherocytosis or sickle cell disease, in which even a brief cessation of erythrocyte production causes a substantial drop in hematocrit. Pure red cell aplasia may also complicate autoimmune diseases, such as systemic lupus erythematosus, rheumatoid arthritis, and Sjögren's syndrome.

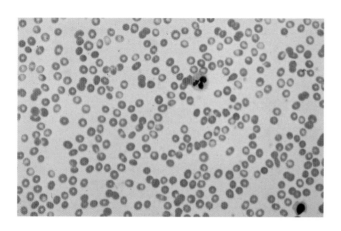

Slide 106. Pure Red Cell Aplasia

In adults, the peripheral blood smear shows a normochromic, normocytic anemia and, despite a diminished hematocrit, the absence of polychromatophilia, indicating deficient release of young cells. The reticulocyte count is extremely low, but the erythropoietin level is appropriately increased for the severity of the anemia. The other cell lines are normal. The bone marrow discloses profound erythroid hypoplasia but normal numbers and maturation of platelet and white cell precursors. In parvovirus infection, giant proerythroblasts with prominent nucleoli may be apparent (see slide 169), and in bone marrow biopsies erythroblasts and erythroid islands are sparse, although proerythroblasts may be numerous. This slide, from a patient with a hematocrit of 7 (!), shows normochromic, normocytic erythrocytes but no polychromatophilia, despite the very low level of circulating red cells. The wide spaces between erythrocytes in most of the smear suggest severe anemia.

ANEMIA WITH DIMORPHISM

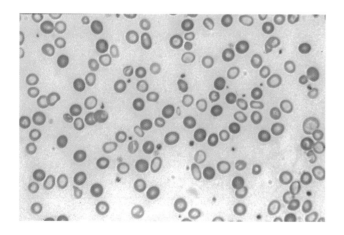

Slide 107. Anemia with Dimorphism

Dimorphism is the presence of two distinct erythrocyte populations of differing sizes, a feature usually appreciated best on low-power examination. Causes include transfusion of normal cells into patients with microcytic or macrocytic anemias, combined iron deficiency and B_{12} or folate deficiency, myelodysplastic syndromes, sideroblastic anemias, and treatment of iron deficiency anemia, in which older microcytic cells coexist with younger normocytic cells. In this slide, from an alcoholic patient with iron deficiency anemia who received a transfusion, normochromic, normocytic erythrocytes intermingle with microcytic, hypochromic cells. A few target and elliptical red cells are present.

Stem-Cell Disorders

APLASTIC ANEMIA

Aplastic anemia refers to bone marrow failure from decreased hematopoietic elements, resulting in peripheral pancytopenia. Sometimes the cause is congenital or inherited, such as Fanconi's syndrome, but most cases are acquired. Aplastic anemia may occur from predictable and dose-dependent physical or chemical damage to the bone marrow, such as radiation, benzene, or cytotoxic agents. It may also arise from idiosyncratic reactions to medications, such as sulfonamides, nonsteroidal anti-inflammatory agents, and anticonvulsants. Infections from certain viruses, including Epstein-Barr virus and human immunodeficiency virus (HIV), are rare causes. Occasional patients, primarily young men, develop the disease after an infectious hepatitis that is seronegative for hepatitis A, B, C, and G viruses. Immune mechanisms, which may govern some cases arising from drugs and infections, probably cause those associated with eosinophilic fasciitis and pregnancy. They certainly produce the aplastic anemia of transfusion-related graft-versus-host disease, which occurs when patients, usually with severely impaired cell-mediated immunity, receive transfusions containing immunocompetent lymphocytes that proliferate and damage the host's tissues, including the bone marrow. It typically occurs a few days to a few weeks after transfusion and has the chief clinical findings of fever, pancytopenia, and a generalized morbilliform eruption, sometimes accompanied by diarrhea, liver enzyme elevations, and hyperbilirubinemia. Although one of the diseases mentioned above is present in some patients, in most cases of aplastic anemia no cause is apparent; many probably originate from immunologic damage to the bone marrow.

The symptoms for which patients initially seek medical attention usually relate to the presence of severe anemia, such as weakness, fatigue, and pallor, or to bleeding related to thrombocytopenia, such as petechiae, purpura, or mucosal hemorrhage from the nose, gingiva, gastrointestinal tract, or uterus. Occasionally, the first manifestation is an infection secondary to severe neutropenia.

On peripheral smear the red cells are normocytic and normochromic; polychromatophilia is absent or rare. The white cells appear normal, but because of neutropenia, lymphocytes typically predominate. The platelets are normal in size and granularity.

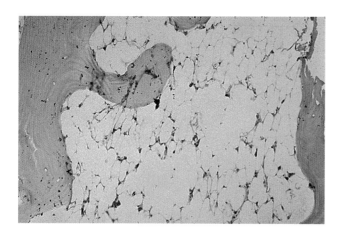

Slide 108. Aplastic Anemia: Bone Marrow Biopsy

In aplastic anemia, bone marrow aspirates are typically difficult to obtain and show fragments primarily containing fat and a few cells. Biopsies disclose increased fat and markedly reduced hematopoiesis. A few areas of cellularity may remain, usually containing normal-appearing cells, but some mild megaloblastic or dysplastic changes may occur. Most of the remaining cells in the bone marrow are lymphocytes, plasma cells, and macrophages. This slide is from a bone marrow biopsy from a patient with severe aplastic anemia. The specimen is virtually devoid of any cellular elements, except for some stroma and hemosiderin-laden macrophages, a sign of iron overload from numerous transfusions.

MYELOPROLIFERATIVE DISORDERS

The myeloproliferative disorders are clonal expansions of marrow stem cells, which cause an excessive production of one or more cell lines. Four diseases are included: polycythemia vera, chronic granulocytic leukemia, idiopathic myelofibrosis (agnogenic myeloid metaplasia), and essential thrombocytosis (thrombocythemia). All may eventuate in acute leukemia; both polycythemia vera and essential thrombocytosis can evolve into myelofibrosis.

Polycythemia Vera

Polycythemia vera is a clonal disorder of the pluripotent hematopoietic stem cell that is characterized by an increased red cell mass, typically with leukocytosis and thrombocytosis as well. Males are affected slightly more than females, and the average age at diagnosis is about 60. Some symptoms, such as headache, paresthesias, dizziness, tinnitus, and visual disturbances, presumably originate from increased blood viscosity caused by the excessive erythrocyte mass. Vascular thromboses, arising from a combination of platelet abnormalities and erythrocytosis, can involve both arterial and venous systems. Common sites of venous occlusion include deep veins of the legs and the splenic, hepatic, portal, cerebral, and mesenteric vessels. Arterial involvement may cause transient ischemic attacks, strokes, myocardial infarctions, and impaired blood flow to the extremities despite palpable pulses, commonly manifested as painful feet and digital ischemia, sometimes producing ulcerations. A distinctive symptom, apparently related to vascular changes caused by thrombocytosis, is erythromelalgia, characterized by erythema, warmth, and a painful burning sensation in the hands or feet that is exacerbated by heat, exercise, or standing and relieved by elevation, cooling, and aspirin therapy.

Hemorrhagic complications also occur, perhaps from impaired platelet function and acquired von Willebrand's syndrome. Common problems are epistaxis or gingival hemorrhage, hematomas, and gastrointestinal bleeding, often associated with peptic ulcers, to which these patients are especially prone. Many patients have generalized itching worsened by contact with water (aquagenic pruritus), probably related to histamine release from basophils. Increased cell production can cause symptoms of hypermetabolism, including sweating and weight loss, and can result in substantial hyperuricemia, present in about 50–70% of patients and often leading to gout. A major finding on examination is a ruddy cyanosis, especially prominent on the nose, ears, neck, cheeks, and lips. The eyes sometimes appear bloodshot because of conjunctival suffusion, and funduscopic examination may reveal distended, tortuous, irregular vessels, with a dark retina and deeply violaceous veins. The mucous membranes of the nose and mouth can have an unusually deep red appearance. Hypertension is common. Hepatic enlargement occurs in about 40% of patients, splenomegaly in approximately 70%.

The hematocrit is elevated, frequently to levels above 60%. Since production of the markedly increased red cell mass commonly causes iron deficiency, the erythrocytes on smear may be hypochromic and microcytic. Polychromatophilia, basophilic stippling, and occasional nucleated red cells are sometimes present. Leukocytosis occurs in about two-thirds of cases, typically with increased basophils, eosinophils, and immature myeloid forms. Thrombocytosis, often with markedly enlarged and bizarrely shaped platelets, occurs in about 50% of patients. Megakaryocyte fragments may be present.

The diagnosis of polycythemia vera depends on finding an increased red cell mass without an alternative explanation, such as chronic hypoxemia or erythropoietin-producing tumors. Features that support polycythemia vera as the cause of erythrocytosis include an arterial oxygen saturation of at least 92% when the patient breathes room air, thrombocytosis, leukocytosis, splenomegaly, low erythropoietin levels, and the ability of bone marrow cells to form erythroid colonies in the absence of exogenous erythropoietin.

Complications of polycythemia vera in addition to those described above are splenic infarcts, postoperative thromboses or hemorrhage in patients with uncontrolled erythrocytosis before surgery, and the development of myeloid metaplasia (myelofibrosis) or acute leukemia. The transition to myeloid metaplasia, which occurs after an average of about 10 years, is heralded by increasing splenomegaly, the appearance of teardrop erythrocytes and leukoery-throblastosis on the blood smear, a decreasing red cell mass, and extensive bone marrow fibrosis. Acute leukemia can develop after myeloid metaplasia, following an intervening phase of a myelodysplastic syndrome, or abruptly, without a transitional step.

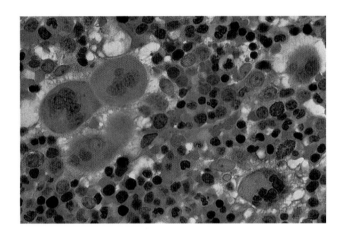

Slide 109. Polycythemia Vera: Bone Marrow Biopsy

In polycythemia vera, the bone marrow aspirate typically discloses erythroid hyperplasia, commonly accompanied by granulocytic and megakaryocytic hyperplasia. Maturation is normal; enlarged megakaryocytes with increased numbers of lobes may be present; and iron stores are commonly depleted or absent. Bone marrow biopsies typically reveal hypercellularity, with increases in all three cell lines. Megakaryocytes are often large and hyperlobulated. Some patients develop significant fibrosis, especially in the presence of substantial megakaryocytic hyperplasia. These patients may enter a "spent phase" characterized by anemia, increasing splenomegaly, and a leukoerythroblastic peripheral blood smear, with many teardrop cells. This slide shows a biopsy with erythroid hyperplasia, evident by the increased numbers of cells with round, regular, central nuclei. Megakaryocytes are increased.

Chronic Myelogenous (Granulocytic) Leukemia

Chronic myelogenous leukemia is a clonal expansion of a pluripotent hematopoietic stem cell, causing marked myeloid hyperplasia, splenomegaly, and leukocytosis that includes immature granulocytes and increased basophils. It accounts for about 15–20% of adult leukemias, has a male to female ratio of about 1.4:1, and typically appears at age 40–60. The predominant symptoms at presentation arise from splenomegaly (left upper quadrant discomfort, early satiety), anemia (fatigue, dyspnea, pallor), and local or systemic manifestations from expansion of the white cell mass (bone pain, sweats, mild fever). About 20–40% of patients are asymptomatic at the time of diagnosis, the disease being discovered on routine physical examination (palpable splenomegaly, present in about one-half of all patients with this disease) or laboratory studies (leukocytosis, anemia, abnormal platelet count). Usually the white cell count is >25,000/mm³ and often exceeds 100,000/mm³, with granulocytes in all stages of maturation present. An increased number of basophils is virtually universal, and eosinophilia is also common. The platelet count is typically raised, sometimes to very high levels, but thrombosis is unusual. Thrombocytopenia at presentation is rare. The serum LDH and uric acid levels are frequently elevated, reflecting increased cell turnover. The leukocyte alkaline phosphatase score is diminished in chronic myelogenous leukemia, unlike in most other disorders causing striking leukocytosis. In 90–95% of cases the Philadelphia chromosome is present, which classically involves a translocation between chromosomes 9 and 22. The abnormal *bcr/abl* gene product from this is detectable by reverse transcriptase polymerase chain reaction (PCR) in more than 95% of cases.

After an average of about 3–4 years, most patients enter an accelerated phase of the disease, with increasing splenomegaly, worsening anemia and thrombocytopenia, rising blasts in the bone marrow and peripheral blood, and bone marrow fibrosis. Some patients have constitutional symptoms of weight loss, fever, and sweats. Extramedullary disease may appear in the lymph nodes, bones, central nervous system, and skin. Masses composed of leukemic cells, previously called chloromas and now labeled granulocytic sarcomas, may form in soft tissues and other sites.

In most cases the disease terminates in "blast crisis," defined by the presence of >30% blasts in the peripheral blood or bone marrow. The hematologic or constitutional features of the accelerated phase described in the preceding paragraph may appear or worsen. The blasts are identifiable by morphologic or immunophenotypic characteristics as myeloblasts in about 50% of cases and as lymphoblasts in 25%; they are undifferentiated in 25%.

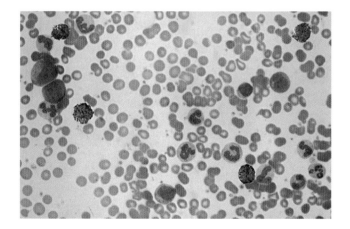

Slide 110. Chronic Granulocytic (Myelogenous) Leukemia: Chronic Phase

In chronic granulocytic leukemia, all stages of the granulocytic series are visible on peripheral smear, but neutrophils, bands, and myelocytes predominate; myeloblasts and promyelocytes are generally <20% of the total cells. Basophils are uniformly increased in number; eosinophils, monocytes, and lymphocytes commonly so. A normocytic, normochromic anemia is usual, and thrombocytosis, sometimes with large platelets, occurs in about 50% of patients. Nucleated red cells are usually visible; other abnormalities sometimes present on the blood smear are hypogranular leukocytes, hypersegmented neutrophils, and megakaryocyte nuclei. In this slide, four basophils are present; the granulocytes range from early forms to mature neutrophils; and platelets are increased in number.

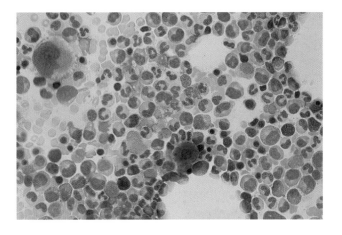

Slide 111. Chronic Granulocytic Leukemia: Bone Marrow Aspirate

The bone marrow aspirate in chronic granulocytic leukemia is markedly hypercellular, with granulocytic hyperplasia but normal maturation. Red cell morphology is normal. Megakaryocytes are numerous but often small, with decreased lobulation. Pseudo-Gaucher cells and sea-blue histiocytes (see also slides 76 and 112) are often present, both being macrophages that contain phagocytized elements produced by the increased bone marrow turnover of cells. This slide shows granulocytic hyperplasia, a small megakaryocyte, and a sea-blue histiocyte in the lower central area.

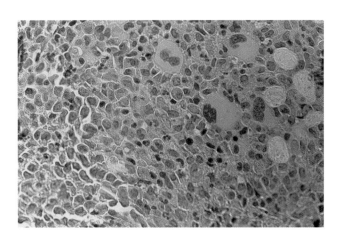

Slide 112. Chronic Granulocytic Leukemia: Bone Marrow Biopsy

In chronic granulocytic leukemia, the bone marrow biopsy demonstrates hypercellularity, primarily of white cell precursors. Megakaryocytes are usually increased as well, although they are smaller than normal and have a decreased number of lobes. Mast cells and plasma cells may be more plentiful than usual, and because of the increased cell turnover, macrophages may contain glycolipids released from the degradation of bone marrow cells. These are pseudo-Gaucher cells, which possess a small eccentric nucleus and an abundant cytoplasm with a crinkled appearance. Bone marrow fibrosis is common in this leukemia and is sometimes severe. In this slide, the marrow shows pronounced granulocytic hyperplasia. Three small megakaryocytes with decreased numbers of lobes are present in one corner, and nearby are five pseudo-Gaucher cells.

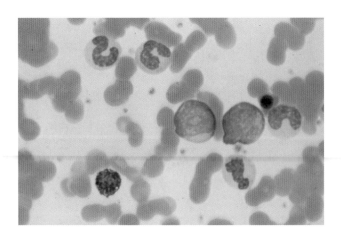

Slide 113. Chronic Granulocytic Leukemia, Blastic Transformation

In "blast crisis" the number of blasts increases and chronic granulocytic leukemia transforms into acute leukemia. This slide, a peripheral smear from a patient with blast crisis, demonstrates neutrophilia, two blasts, a nucleated red cell, and a basophil.

Idiopathic Myelofibrosis (Agnogenic Myeloid Metaplasia)

Idiopathic myelofibrosis is a clonal disorder of hematopoietic stem cells characterized by splenomegaly, extramedullary hematopoiesis, and marrow fibrosis, thought to develop from stimulation of fibroblasts by growth factors produced by megakaryocytes. The disease occurs primarily in older people, with no sex preference. The average age at diagnosis is about 60 years. Excessive radiation exposure is a risk factor, but in most patients no predisposing condition is apparent. About 20% of patients are asymptomatic and the disease is discovered on routine physical examination or laboratory studies. The most common symptoms arise from (1) anemia, (2) splenomegaly, or (3) hypermetabolism from marked cell turnover. Those related to anemia include fatigue, weakness, and dyspnea. Enlargement of the spleen may cause left upper quadrant discomfort, diarrhea from splenic compression of the intestines, and early satiety from pressure on the stomach. Symptoms due to hypermetabolism include weight loss, night sweats, and fever or problems related to hyperuricemia—gout or urinary tract obstruction from urate stones. Another presenting feature may be bleeding caused by thrombocytopenia. On examination, splenomegaly is universal and may be massive. Hepatomegaly occurs in about 50–70% and lymph node enlargement in 10–20%. Cutaneous petechiae and purpura from thrombocytopenia may be present, and occasionally extramedullary hematopoiesis in the skin is apparent as red to violaceous nodules, plaques, and papules. Ascites can occur from extramedullary hematopoiesis affecting the peritoneal surface or from portal hypertension related to hepatic involvement or increased blood flow from the spleen to the liver.

Anemia, present in most patients, results from several factors: ineffective hematopoiesis, dilution of erythrocytes due to an expanded plasma volume, and shortened red cell survival. The life span of erythrocytes can be diminished by diverse mechanisms, including destruction in the spleen, red cell autoantibodies, and a sensitivity to complement identical to that seen in paroxysmal nocturnal hemoglobinuria. The white cell count is elevated in about 50%, decreased in about 25%. Thrombocytosis, sometimes to marked levels, occurs in approximately 50% of patients, but with disease progression, thrombocytopenia becomes common. Other frequent laboratory abnormalities include increased serum LDH levels, hyperuricemia, and elevated transaminase, bilirubin, and alkaline phosphatase levels.

Complications of agnogenic myeloid metaplasia comprise splenic infarcts or hematomas, progressive splenic enlargement, and pain in the spleen and bones, which may demonstrate myelosclerosis on radiographic studies. Esophageal varices with gastrointestinal hemorrhage may develop because of portal hypertension that originates from portal or hepatic vein thromboses, hepatic extramedullary hematopoiesis, or increased blood flow from the spleen to the liver. Tumors composed of extramedullary hematopoietic tissue can form in any organ, causing enlargement, bleeding, fluid formation, or compression of adjacent normal tissue. These may develop in the dura, producing symptoms and signs related to the brain, cranial nerves, or spinal cord. Involvement of the serosal surfaces can lead to increased fluid in the pleura, pericardium, or peritoneal cavities. The presence of these tumors in the urinary tract can cause obstruction or hematuria. About 10–20% of patients with idiopathic myelofibrosis eventually develop acute myelogenous leukemia.

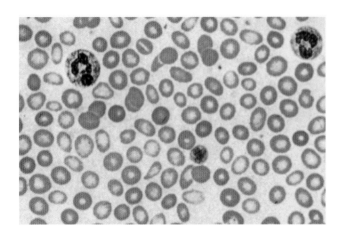

Slide 114. Idiopathic Myelofibrosis (Agnogenic Myeloid Metaplasia)

In this disorder, the peripheral blood smear discloses leukoerythroblastosis (the presence of nucleated red cells and immature myeloid cells) and teardrop erythrocytes (dacrocytes) in almost all patients. The dacryocytes partly originate in the spleen, since they decrease following splenectomy. Other red cell abnormalities include fragments, numerous polychromatophilic cells, ovalocytes, elliptocytes, and basophilic stippling. Neutrophils whose nuclei are hypersegmented or hyposegmented (acquired Pelger-Huët anomaly) and occasional blasts may be visible. Increased basophils and eosinophils are common. Large platelets and intact or fragmented megakaryocytes are characteristic. In this slide, poikilocytosis and anisocytosis are obvious. Two neutrophils are present, reflecting the leukocytosis seen in this patient. A teardrop cell is present in the lower center, and a giant platelet sits near it.

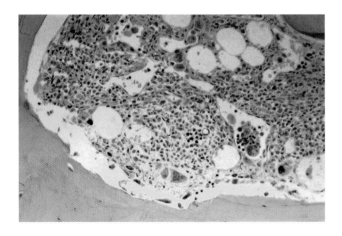

Slide 115. Idiopathic Myelofibrosis: Bone Marrow Biopsy

Because of the bone marrow fibrosis in this disorder, aspirates may be difficult or impossible to obtain (the so-called dry tap), but early in the disease they may show hypercellularity affecting all cell lines. In the first stages of the disease, bone marrow biopsies may also show hypercellularity, usually with a predominance of megakaryocytes displaying pleomorphic nuclei and a wide range of sizes. As this disorder progresses, fibrosis increases, and the hematopoietic cells diminish. This slide of a biopsy specimen shows hypercellularity with numerous megakaryocytes. The sinuses are dilated, and in several intrasinusoidal areas hematopoiesis is occurring, most prominently in the right lower corner.

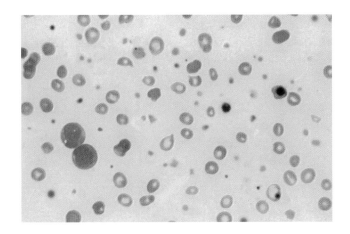

Slide 116. Idiopathic Myelofibrosis: Leukemic Transformation

About 10–20% of cases of idiopathic myelofibrosis terminate in acute leukemia, usually myelogenous. In this slide, two blasts are present in the left lower corner. Other findings include a nucleated red cell, thrombocytosis, some large platelets, a Howell-Jolly body in an erythrocyte in the right lower corner, and a teardrop cell in the center.

Essential Thrombocythemia

Essential thrombocythemia (thrombocytosis) is a clonal disorder affecting a multipotent hematopoietic stem cell that results in megakaryocyte hyperplasia and an elevated platelet count in the blood. The median age at diagnosis is about 50–60 years, and the disease is slightly more common in women. Many patients are asymptomatic, the disorder being discovered on a routine blood test. Most symptoms develop from vessel occlusion or abnormal reactivity of the small or large vasculature; these include headaches, dizziness, visual disturbances, distal paresthesias, transient ischemic attacks, and skin lesions. A distinctive finding, present in about 5% of cases, is erythromelalgia, characterized by erythema, warmth, and a painful burning sensation in the hands or feet that is exacerbated by heat, exercise, or standing and relieved by elevation, cooling, and aspirin. Other cutaneous findings include evidence of bleeding, (hematomas, ecchymoses, petechiae, purpura), ischemia (ulcerations, gangrene), or abnormal patterns of blood flow (livedo reticularis, acrocyanosis). Thrombotic episodes primarily affect the arteries, including those of the cerebral, coronary, renal, and peripheral vasculature. Venous thromboses may form in several locations, such as the hepatic, portal, ophthalmic, intestinal, cerebral, and leg veins. Major hemorrhage is less common but can occur in the soft tissues, joints, and gastrointestinal tract. Splenomegaly is present in about 20–50% of patients but is usually moderate and nonprogressive; hepatomegaly is detectable in about 20%.

Usually the platelet count exceeds 1 million/mm³, and the cells are often large, but may vary considerably in size and shape. Megakaryocyte fragments are commonly visible. Immature myeloid precursors and nucleated red cells can be present, usually in small numbers. The hematocrit is typically normal to slightly diminished, the white cell count is often mildly increased, and basophilia and eosinophilia may occur. The serum uric acid and LDH levels are often elevated. The bone marrow aspirate and biopsy usually demonstrate increased numbers of large, normally lobulated megakaryocytes. On biopsies, the megakaryocytes often appear in clusters and with pleomorphic nuclei. The reticulin is often increased, as are the numbers of granulocyte and erythrocyte precursors.

Because several disorders can cause thrombocytosis, including other myeloproliferative and myelodysplastic syndromes, iron deficiency, inflammatory or malignant diseases, infections, and asplenia, the diagnosis of essential thrombocythemia depends on excluding these causes. Widely accepted criteria are (1) a platelet count > 600,000/mm³; (2) a hematocrit < 40 or a normal red cell mass [to exclude polycythemia vera]; (3) stainable iron in marrow, normal serum ferritin, or normal mean corpuscular volume [to exclude iron deficiency]; (4) no Philadelphia chromosome or *bcr/abl* gene rearrangement [to exclude chronic granulocytic leukemia]; (5) absent collagen fibrosis on marrow biopsy or constituting less than one-third of the biopsy area without both marked splenomegaly and leukoerythroblastic reaction [to exclude idiopathic myelofibrosis]; (6) no cytogenetic or morphologic evidence for a myelodysplastic syndrome; and (7) no cause for reactive thrombocytosis.

Most patients with essential thrombocythemia have a normal life expectancy, with the commonest cause of death being thrombotic episodes. In some patients the disease transforms into another myeloproliferative disorder (polycythemia vera, agnogenic myeloid metaplasia), a myelodysplastic disease, or acute leukemia.

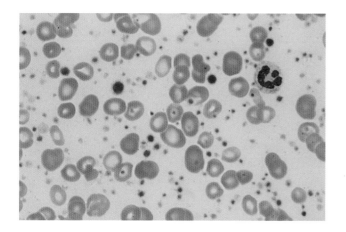

Slide 117. Essential Thrombocythemia

In this disease the platelets are often giant, have bizarre shapes, and demonstrate increased or decreased granules. Neutrophilia may be present, as may nucleated red cells and immature granulocytes (leukoerythroblastosis). Poikilocytosis is frequent. This slide shows a remarkable increase in the number of platelets, which are of varying sizes and granulation.

MYELODYSPLASTIC SYNDROMES

The myelodysplastic syndromes are disorders arising from the clonal expansion of an abnormal myeloid precursor in which the marrow is usually hypercellular but the maturation is abnormal (dysplastic), leading to death of the cells in the marrow (ineffective hematopoiesis) and peripheral cytopenias in one or more blood cell lines. Some cases occur from prior exposure to cytotoxic agents or radiation therapy, and in these patients marrow hypoplasia and increased reticulin fibrosis are common. Most cases of myelodysplasia, however, arise as an apparently primary problem, predominantly in people over 60 years of age. About one-half of patients are asymptomatic, their disorder being discovered on a routine blood cell count. Symptoms usually relate to anemia, such as fatigue and dyspnea, but some patients have recurrent infections from neutropenia or bleeding problems from thrombocytopenia. Palpable splenomegaly is present in a small number of patients, except in chronic myelomonocytic leukemia, where it occurs in 30–50% of cases. A complication is Sweet's syndrome, a febrile disorder characterized by cutaneous plaques and nodules caused by neutrophilic infiltration of the dermis.

Many patients have cytogenetic abnormalities, primarily deletions of various parts of chromosomes, but translocations and gains or losses of whole chromosomes sometimes occur. The most common type of cytogenetic abnormality, usually presenting as refractory anemia, is deletion of the long arm of chromosome 5 (5q − syndrome). It typically occurs in middle-aged to elderly women who have a macrocytic anemia, normal platelet counts, and large, hypolobular megakaryocytes.

Common to the myelodysplastic syndromes are cells in the circulating blood and bone marrow demonstrating abnormal maturation. Evidence of impaired *erythropoiesis* consists of anemia, present in nearly all cases, and abnormalities on peripheral smear, such as macrocytosis, anisocytosis, basophilic stippling, and Pappenheimer bodies. Poikilocytosis is typical and includes ovalocytes, stomatocytes, acanthocytes, elliptocytes, red cell fragments, target cells, and teardrop cells. Sometimes nucleated red cells are visible, and they may demonstrate abnormalities of maturation, such as megaloblastic or multilobed nuclei. Occasional findings include microcytosis and polychromasia. Features of altered erythropoiesis in the bone marrow are hyperplasia, multinuclear fragments, bizarre nuclear shapes, pyknotic nuclei, mitoses, basophilic stippling, internuclear bridging, and abnormal chromatin, either dense or fine, in a cell whose cytoplasm reflects a stage of maturity different from the nuclei. On iron stain the stores are usually increased, and erythroblasts may demonstrate an increased number of ferritin granules (more than four), sometimes comprising more than one-third of the nuclear rim (ringed sideroblasts).

On peripheral smear, evidence of abnormal *granulopoiesis* includes granulocytopenia, Döhle bodies, and neutrophils with hypersegmented, ringed, or bizarre-shaped nuclei. Another finding is decreased or absent cytoplasmic granules in neutrophils and eosinophils, the demonstration of which requires a very careful examination under oil immersion. The nuclei of neutrophils are often hypolobulated and have dense chromatin clumping. Some have a single lobe, some are bilobed with a thin connecting strand of chromatin, and some appear peanut-shaped. Immature cells, including blasts, with or without Auer rods, may be visible. Eosinophils and basophils can also have hypogranulation and abnormal lobulation. Sometimes the number of monocytes is elevated, and promonocytes are detectable. In the bone marrow, granulocytic hyperplasia is usual, often with increased numbers of blasts. Megaloblastic changes can occur, and in bone marrow sections, the granulocyte precursors may be present centrally rather than in their usual paratrabecular position, a phenomenon called atypical localization of immature precursors (ALIP).

Evidence of abnormal *thrombopoiesis* on peripheral blood smears includes thrombocytopenia, giant platelets, and those with decreased or absent granules. In bone marrow specimens the megakaryocytes demonstrate either reduced size (micromegakaryocyte), defined as smaller than promyelocytes, or separate nuclear lobulations.

A group of hematologists from France, America, and Great Britain (the FAB group) has used the peripheral blood and bone marrow findings to define five types of myelodysplasia (FAB classification): *refractory anemia* (about 30% of cases), *refractory anemia with ring sideroblasts* (25%), *refractory anemia with excess blasts* (20%), *refractory anemia with excess blasts in transition* (10%), and *chronic myelomonocytic leukemia* (15%). The diagnostic criteria depend on evaluating both peripheral smears and bone marrow samples, in conjunction with cytogenetic analysis. Especially important is enumerating the number of blasts in both types of specimens and ringed sideroblasts on iron stains of bone marrow samples. For the FAB classifications of both the myelodysplastic syndromes and the acute myeloid leukemias, blasts in the bone marrow are calculated as a percentage of the total nucleated cells or, if erythroblasts constitute 50% or more of these cells, then as a percentage of the nonerythroid nucleated cells, excluding lymphocytes, plasma cells, mast cells, and macrophages. Once bone marrow blasts are 30% or more, leukemia, not myelodysplasia, is present. The World Health Organization (WHO) classification of myelodysplasia includes additional morphologic (such as multilineage versus single lineage dysplasia) and cytogenetic (5q-syndrome) parameters in subtyping this disease. The WHO classification eliminates the category of refractory anemia with excess blasts in transition and instead recognizes myelodysplasia with greater than 20% blasts as acute myeloid leukemia.

In using the FAB system to differentiate the myelodysplasias, the first step is to examine the blood and bone marrow for blasts. According to this classification, refractory anemia with excess blasts in transformation occurs when the peripheral blast count reaches 5%, the bone marrow blast percentage is 20–30%, or blasts with Auer rods are present in blood or bone marrow. In patients without these features, the next step is to enumerate the monocytes in the blood, and if they exceed 1,000/mm^3 (1 × 10^9/L), chronic myelomonocytic leukemia is present. In patients without these features, further classification rests on the number of blasts and ringed sideroblasts. With peripheral blasts of 1% or bone marrow blasts of 5%, the diagnosis is refractory anemia with excess blasts. If these features are absent but ringed sideroblasts account for more than 15% of the erythroblasts, the diagnosis is refractory anemia with ringed sideroblasts. The remaining cases are classified as refractory anemia (or refractory cytopenia when anemia is absent but thrombocytopenia or neutropenia is present).

In hematologic practice, the diagnosis of myelodysplastic syndrome is made (1) clinically, as a diagnosis of last resort for primary bone marrow-based cytopenia(s), (2) pathologically, or (3) cytogenetically. In most cases of myelodysplastic syndrome the diagnosis rests on a combination of the above. It is difficult to standardize criteria for making any diagnosis based purely on a cytological basis, but it is still useful to follow some universal guidelines for what is meant by "dysplastic" and how one comes to make a morphologic diagnosis of primary myelodysplasia. Well-preserved and adequately stained marrow spicules are essential. A history of (1) previous exposure to myelotoxic agents (including chemotherapy, radiation, and other toxins) or (2) nutritional deficiencies (vitamin B_{12} and folate) are causes of secondary myelodysplastic syndrome to be excluded before considering a diagnosis of primary myelodysplastic syndrome. A useful rule for making a morphologic diagnosis of myelodysplastic syndrome is finding dysplastic changes in at least two out of three hematopoietic lineages (myeloid, megakaryocytic, and erythroid). In the early stages of myelodysplastic syndrome and in most cases at the time of initial diagnosis, dysplastic changes are almost never found in all the cells of a particular lineage but only in a minority. Accordingly, the examiner should carefully assess many marrow cells from all three lineages when evaluating a marrow specimen for myelodysplastic syndrome. The most characteristic dysplastic changes in the myeloid line, best seen in the peripheral smear, include hypolobulated nuclei and hypogranular cytoplasm. Characteristic dysplastic changes in the erythroid lineage, seen in the marrow, are asymmetric multinucleation, irregular nuclear contours, other bizarre nuclear contour abnormalities, and ringed sideroblasts with iron staining. Micromegakaryocytes (smaller than a promyelocyte) and forms displaying clearly separate nuclear lobulations are recognized dysplastic findings in megakaryocytes.

Many patients with myelodysplastic syndrome eventually develop acute leukemia, nearly always myelogenous, which may appear suddenly or may gradually evolve over several weeks to months. The likelihood varies according to the type of myelodysplastic syndrome present; the descending order of risk is refractory anemia with excess blasts in transition, refractory anemia with excess blasts, chronic myelomonocytic leukemia, refractory anemia with ringed sideroblasts, and refractory anemia. The chance of developing leukemia is quite high in the first three types, much lower in the latter two.

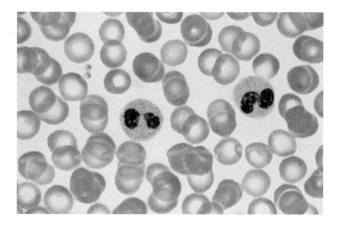

Slide 118. Myelodysplasia: Pseudo-Pelger-Huët Cell

A common finding in the myelodysplastic and myelo-proliferative syndromes is the pseudo-Pelger-Huët cell. It consists of bilobed neutrophils, typically with a small bridge connecting the two lobes. The cells resemble those in the autosomal dominant disorder of the Pelger-Huët anomaly, but in the acquired form, the number of affected neutrophils is generally lower, and additional dysplastic features are present in the granulocytes or other cell lines. In this slide a pseudo-Pelger-Huët cell is seen on the left. A thin string of chromatin connects its two lobes (pince-nez appearance; see slide 24). The white cell on the right is a normal band with a twisted nucleus.

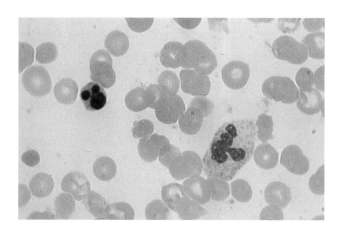

Slide 119. Myelodysplastic Syndromes: Peripheral Blood

This slide, from a patient with chronic myelomono-cytic leukemia, shows a nucleated erythrocyte that is dysplastic in having a lobulated nucleus. The white cell is a bizarre, hypersegmented monocyte. Platelets are diminished.

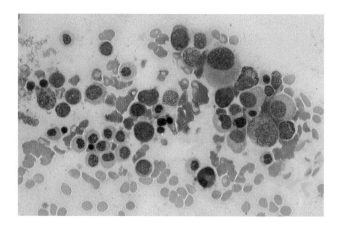

Slide 120. Myelodysplastic Syndromes: Bone Marrow Aspirate

Despite the decreased numbers of red cells, platelets, and white cells in the peripheral smear in these disorders, the aspirate is usually hypercellular. Dysplasia in the hematopoietic lines is the most important finding. In this slide, from a patient with chemotherapy-induced myelodysplasia, the megakaryocyte in the right upper area is small and shows hypolobulation and sparse, poorly granulated cytoplasm. A cluster of dysplastic, hypogranular, and hypolobulated myeloid precursors with abnormally condensed nuclei appears in the lower left. Myeloid maturation is absent.

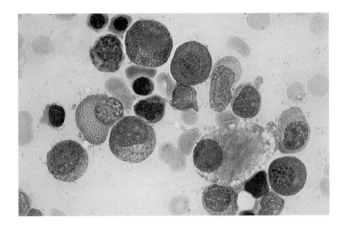

Slide 121. Myelodysplasia: Bone Marrow Aspirate

This bone marrow aspirate illustrates dysplasia in several cells. On the left of the slide is a cell with refractile granules that partially cover a single nucleus. This is a dysplastic, unilobular eosinophil whose granules are less intense than usual. The cell with abundant vacuolated cytoplasm on the right is a dysplastic micromegakaryocyte with only a single-lobed nucleus.

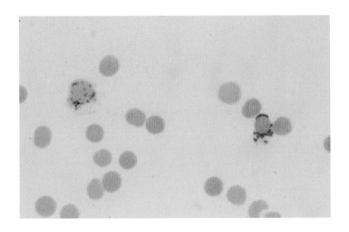

Slide 122. Refractory Anemia with Ringed Sideroblasts: Bone Marrow Aspirate, Iron Stain

In this disease, the peripheral smear usually demonstrates macrocytic red cells, but often with a smaller population of microcytic, hypochromic cells—a dimorphic anemia. Basophilic stippling, Pappenheimer bodies, and nucleated red cells may be present. The bone marrow aspirate typically discloses erythroid hyperplasia with dysplastic changes. The other cell lines are usually normal, and blasts are less than 5%. On iron stain, ringed sideroblasts constitute more than 15% of the nucleated red cells. Ringed sideroblasts have iron granules arranged in a ring around the nucleus rather than in a random distribution throughout the cytoplasm (see slide 62). This slide shows two ringed sideroblasts.

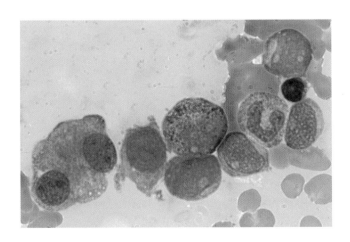

Slide 123. Refractory Anemia with Excess Blasts: Bone Marrow Aspirate

In this disorder, blasts represent 1–5% of the peripheral white cells or 5–20% of the bone marrow cells. On peripheral smear, in addition to the presence of blasts, pancytopenia is common, and dysplastic features affect the different cell types. The bone marrow aspirate shows hypercellularity, with dysplasia usually present in all lines, and the defining increase in blasts. In this slide, at least four of the cells are blasts. At the left is a small, dysplastic megakaryocyte with separated nuclear lobules.

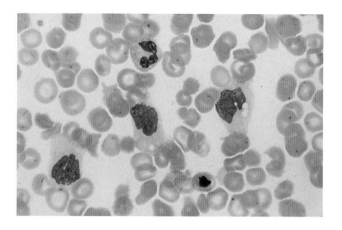

Slide 124. Chronic Myelomonocytic Leukemia

This diagnosis requires a monocyte count of $>1 \times 10^9/L$ ($>1,000/mm^3$), with up to 20% blasts in the bone marrow and no more than 5% blasts in the peripheral blood. In the bone marrow promonocytes are often increased, and neutrophils are frequently numerous on the peripheral smear. The monocytes often appear normal, but some have bizarre shapes or hypersegmented nuclei and increased cytoplasmic basophilia. Dysplasia occurs in the other cell lines as well. This slide shows a dysplastic nucleated red cell with a pyknotic nucleus, displaying irregular borders and three atypical monocytes, reflecting the profound peripheral monocytosis in this patient. Howell-Jolly bodies are present in several red cells.

White Cell Disorders

LEUKEMIAS

Acute Leukemias

The proliferation of undifferentiated bone marrow cells of either lymphoid or myeloid origin produces acute lymphocytic (ALL) or acute myeloid leukemia (AML), respectively. Acute leukemia represents a clonal expansion of abnormal immature cells that often have diagnostically significant chromosomal abnormalities such as translocations. At the time of presentation, leukemia cells have usually replaced the marrow cavity and spilled out into the blood. The term *acute* with regard to leukemia no longer denotes a rapid fatal outcome but refers to the undifferentiated state of the leukemia cells. In fact, most patients present with nonspecific symptoms such as fatigue, lethargy, and weight loss. Older people with acute leukemia may complain of dyspnea, angina, and dizziness related to anemia. Approximately one-third of patients have serious infections at the time of diagnosis, and, with the exception of AML-M3, rarely do serious bleeding problems pose a problem at that point.

Acute leukemia is slightly more common in white men and has been correlated with high socioeconomic status. AML, which constitutes approximately 80% of all acute leukemias in adults, is a disease of the elderly, with its incidence rising after age 50. ALL, on the other hand, occurs primarily in children and young adults, with a median age in adults ranging from 25 to 40 years. Risk factors for acute leukemia include previous exposure to ionizing radiation, benzene, and certain classes of chemotherapeutic drugs, including alkylating agents and topoisomerase II-inhibitors. Patients with Down syndrome are at increased risk of developing acute leukemia. Other predisposing conditions include rare hereditary chromosome breakage (Bloom's syndrome and Fanconi's anemia) and immunodeficiency (Bruton-type X-linked agammaglobulinemia and hereditary ataxia-telangiectasia) syndromes.

At the time of presentation, the peripheral blood usually shows anemia, neutropenia, and thrombocytopenia, although the total white cell count is highly variable. Circulating blasts are apparent in the peripheral blood in approximately 80% of cases. So-called aleukemic leukemia, a term used when circulating blasts are absent, is slightly more common in AML than ALL. Important features to assess in the peripheral blood of newly diagnosed acute leukemia include (1) signs of intravascular coagulation (which suggest acute promyelocytic leukemia, AML-M3), such as a microangiopathic picture with severe anisopoikilocytosis, microcytes, red cell fragments, schistocytes, and profound thrombocytopenia; (2) hyperleukocytosis (especially in AML-3); (3) signs of underlying myelodysplasia, such as hypolobulated and hypogranular neutrophils; and (4) Auer rods in circulating blasts.

After a complete history and physical examination, all patients with acute leukemia should have slides of their peripheral blood and representative bone marrow specimens scrutinized. In addition, all those with ALL and AML with monocytic differentiation (AML-M4 and AML-M5) should undergo lumbar puncture to examine the cerebrospinal fluid (CSF) for the presence of blasts. A diagnosis of acute leukemia rests upon demonstrating an increased number of immature hematopoietic cells and then assigning a particular lineage, generally either myeloid or lymphoid, to the abnormal leukemic cell population. The most widely used classification is that originally proposed by the French-American-British (FAB) Cooperative Group in 1976 (*Br J Haematol* 1976;33:452–8). The World Health Organization has incorporated much of the FAB classification into an expanded version (*J Clin Oncol* 1999;17:3835–49). A diagnosis of acute leukemia is made after examining Wright's- or Wright's-Giemsa stained bone marrow aspirate smears and peripheral blood along with a hematoxylin-eosin (H&E)-stained clot section and biopsy. In addition, in all newly diagnosed cases of acute leukemia, cytogenetic analysis and histochemical and flow immunophenotyping should be done on the cells.

The diagnosis of acute leukemia is usually not subtle. Bone marrow examination most commonly reveals a hypercellular specimen with sheets of blasts. The normal marrow constituents—the erythroid, maturing myeloid, and megakaryocytes—are usually markedly diminished in number. Occasionally, most often in cases of high-grade myelodysplasia (refractory anemia with excess blasts), the marrow exhibits atypical morphological features. In these cases, overall marrow cellularity may be low, the erythroid series markedly increased, populations of atypical or dysplastic megakaryocytes expanded, and extensive marrow fibrosis seen. In addition, so-called hypoplastic variants of acute leukemia, usually AML, exist, characterized by low total marrow cellularity but relatively high numbers of blasts. Rarely, acute leukemia can arise from an extramedullary focus, usually a blast crisis complicating a preexisting myeloproliferative syndrome, and marrow samples are nonrepresentative.

Nearly always, a diagnosis of acute leukemia can be made by recognizing increased blasts and determining the lineage by histochemical and/or surface phenotype studies. A diagnosis of de novo acute leukemia requires that at least 30% of the total nucleated bone marrow cells be blasts, with three exceptions. If the marrow displays displastic erythroid hyperplasia (erythroblasts ≥ 50% of total cells) and if ≥30% of nonerythroid cells are blasts, a diagnosis of AML with erythroid differentiation (AML-M6) is made. Another exception is in myelodysplastic syndrome (MDS) when myeloblasts are $\geq 20\%$ of total marrow cells. This condition, formerly called "refractory anemia with excess blasts-in-transformation" (RAEB-T) is now recognized as AML. The third exception is acute promyelocytic leukemia (AML-M3), in which abnormal promyelocytes rather than increased blasts constitute the majority of marrow cells. A blast is defined morphologically as a cell that is medium to large in size, usually has a high nuclear:cytoplasm ratio, possesses an open chromatin pattern with or without nucleoli, and typically has sparse basophilic-staining cytoplasm. Fine azurophilic (bright red/purple) cytoplasmic granulation is sometimes present in blasts (so-called type II blasts). Unless it contains an Auer rod, a blast cannot be classified as either myeloid or lymphoid without ancillary histochemical or phenotypic studies. Once increased blasts are recognized, the origin—either lymphoid or myeloid—must be determined to make a diagnosis of ALL or AML, respectively. The recommended approach is to first rule in AML by showing positive cytoplasmic staining with myeloid granule–specific stains such as myeloperoxidase (or Sudan Black) and monocytic-specific stain such as α-naphthyl acetate esterase. If $\leq 3\%$ of the blasts are positive with the myeloid granule–specific stain, immunophenotyping by flow cytometry is recommended. Since blasts of one type of AML, AML with minimal evidence of myeloid differentiation (AML-M0), are negative with these myeloid granule–specific stains, negative staining does not exclude a diagnosis of AML. For this reason, flow immunophenotyping is indicated to rule out AML-M0 if the myeloid-specific histochemical stains are negative.

Acute Myeloid Leukemias

The FAB classification of acute myeloid leukemias (sometimes called acute nonlymphocytic leukemia, or ANLL) depends largely on a 500-cell differential count of a bone marrow specimen. The FAB classification includes seven types of acute myeloid leukemia defined by the nature of the blast cells; usually these cells are also present on the peripheral blood smear, allowing a presumptive diagnosis to be made. This system recognizes three types of blasts. Type I are myeloblasts lacking cytoplasmic granules but possessing prominent nucleoli, a central nucleus, and uncondensed chromatin patterns. Type II blasts resemble type I cells and retain a central nucleus but have a few primary (azurophilic) cytoplasmic granules. Type III cells have more than 20 azurophilic cytoplasmic granules but do not display a Golgi zone, which is characteristic of promyelocytes.

In addition to the abnormalities in white cells, anemia and thrombocytopenia are common, as are morphologic changes in the erythrocytes and platelets on the peripheral smear. Anisocytosis, poikilocytosis, basophilic stippling, and nucleated red cells are often present among the erythrocytes. Leukemic cells may sometimes ingest red cells (erythrophagocytosis). In the platelet series, giant or agranular platelets and circulating micromegakaryocytes may be visible.

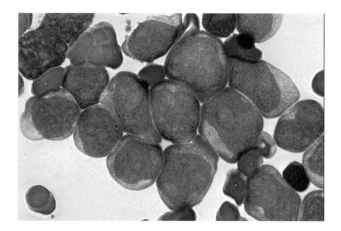

Slide 125. Acute Myeloblastic Leukemia Without Maturation (M1): Bone Marrow Aspirate

In M1, blasts constitute at least 90% of the nucleated cells of the bone marrow. The blast is usually a medium to large cell with a round or oval nucleus containing one or more nucleoli. The cytoplasm may possess a few granules, vacuoles, and Auer rods, which are red, needle-like structures thought to be coalescences of primary granules. About 15–20% of acute myeloid leukemias are M1. This slide shows the relatively uniform appearance of the blasts, which have an "open" (very fine reticulated) chromatin pattern, one to two prominent nucleoli, and scant to moderate amounts of basophilic cytoplasm.

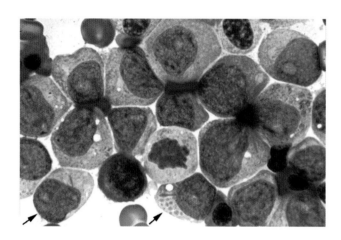

Slide 126. Acute Myeloblastic Leukemia with Maturation (M2): Bone Marrow Aspirate

In M2, the same kinds of blasts are present as in M1, but they account for 30–89% of the nucleated cells in the bone marrow, with differentiation of at least 10% of the remaining cells into granulocytic series (promyelocytes to neutrophils) and less than 20% of the nonerythroid cells being in the monocytic line. This subtype constitutes about 20% of acute myeloid leukemias. In this slide, the preeminent cells are myeloblasts. The *arrows* point to two of the myeloblasts that contain Auer rods in the cytoplasm. Many of the blasts have eccentric nuclei with closed chromatin and ample cytoplasm with fine gray granulation, features indicative of myeloid maturation. The fact that these more mature granulocytes constituted >10% of the white cells allowed the diagnosis of M2 to be made in this case.

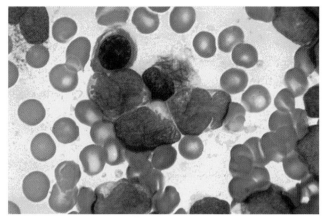

Slide 127. Acute Hypergranular Promyelocytic Leukemia (M3): Bone Marrow Aspirate

In this leukemia, the blasts are usually <30% of nucleated bone marrow cells, but the typical morphology of the predominant cell allows the diagnosis to be made with confidence. The abnormal promyelo-cyte is larger than a normal myeloblast; has an oval, kidney-shaped, folded, or bilobed nucleus; and possesses a cytoplasm replete with large, sometimes giant, red or purplish granules that may obscure the nucleus. The cytoplasm commonly has abundant Auer rods as well. A variant form, M3V, has cells with reniform, lobulated, or convoluted nuclei and cytoplasm that may be either agranular or sparsely but finely granulated. These two forms of M3 constitute about 10% of acute myeloid leukemias. This slide shows promyelocytes with folded and bilobed nuclei. The four in the center of the slide with impressive accumulations of Auer rods are sometimes called "faggot cells," because their contents resemble a bundle of sticks. A single erythroid precursor lies above the promyelocytes. Most cases of M3 and M3V AML have a balanced reciprocal translocation between chromosomes 15 and 17, t(15;17)(q22;q21), that can be detected by cytogenetic fluorescence in situ hybridization (FISH) analyses.

Slide 128. Acute Myelomonocytic Leukemia (M4): Peripheral Blood

In this disorder, blasts constitute 30–89% of the nucleated bone marrow cells. The granulocytic compo-

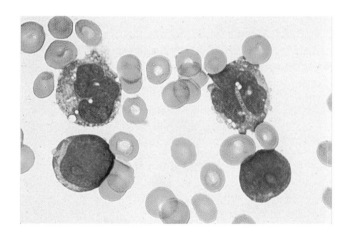

nent (including myeloblasts) and the monocytic component (monoblasts, promonocytes, monocytes) each account for at least 20% of the bone marrow cells. In the peripheral blood, monocytes are often very numerous, reaching levels of more than 5×10^9/L (5,000/mm³). The predominant cells are monoblasts and promonocytes. The monoblast is a large cell whose round or convoluted nucleus has lacy chromatin and one or more nucleoli, which may be large; the cytoplasm is ample, basophilic, often vacuolated, and sometimes granulated. Auer rods are occasionally present. In promonocytes as compared to monoblasts, the nucleoli are smaller, the nuclei are often indented, the cytoplasm has more numerous granules, and its color is more basophilic. M4 accounts for about 15–20% of acute myeloid leukemia. This slide from a peripheral smear shows two monocytes and two blasts, reflecting the dual populations of blasts, myeloid and monocytic, typical for this subtype of AML.

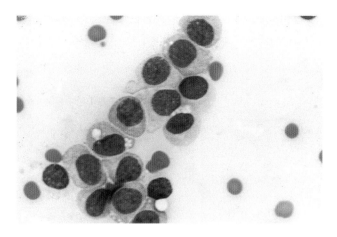

Slide 129. Acute Monocytic Leukemia (M5): Bone Marrow Aspirate

In M5, blasts constitute at least 30% of the bone marrow's nucleated cells, and the monocytic component is at least 80% of the nonerythroid cells. M5 is subdivided into M5a (acute monoblastic leukemia), if monoblasts account for at least 80% of the bone marrow monocytic component, and M5b, if they are less than that percentage. This slide, from a patient with M5, shows numerous monoblasts with lacy chromatin, round or oval nuclei, nucleoli, and gray cytoplasm.

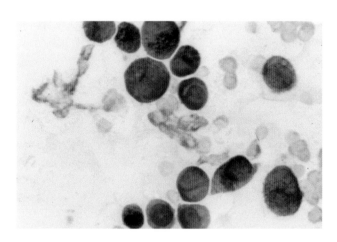

Slide 130. Acute Monocytic Leukemia (M5): Bone Marrow Aspirate, Esterase Stain

Cytochemical stains can confirm the cell type of this leukemia, since the monocyte and its precursors react with the nonspecific esterase stains, α-naphthyl acetate esterase or α-naphthyl butyrate esterase. In this slide, the red material in the cytoplasm of the cells indicates a positive reaction for nonspecific esterases.

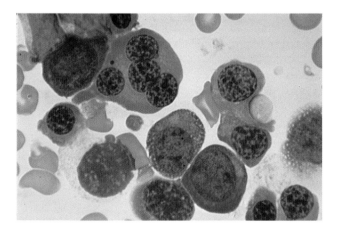

Slide 131. Acute Myeloid Leukemia with Prominent Erythroid Differentiation (M6): Bone Marrow Aspirate

In M6 (erythroleukemia), dysplastic erythroid precursors must constitute at least 50% of the nucleated cells in the bone marrow and granulocytic blasts must account for at least 30% of the nonerythroid cells or at least 20% of nonerythroid cells using the FAB or WHO classifications, respectively. The erythroblasts usually show substantial dysplasia, including cytoplasmic vacuolization, bizarre nuclear features, multinuclearity, megaloblastic changes, and karyorrhexis (rupture of the nucleus). M6 represents about 3–4% of acute myeloid leukemias. This slide shows several erythroblasts, two with multinuclearity, two with cytoplasmic vacuoles, and some with megaloblastic changes, characterized by large nuclei with loose chromatin in cells with polychromatophilic cytoplasm.

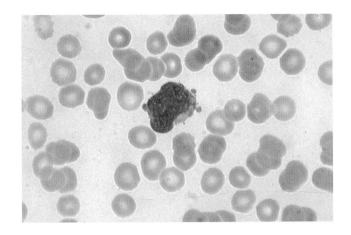

Slide 132. Acute Megakaryoblastic Leukemia (M7)

In M7, blasts constitute at least 30% of the bone marrow nucleated cells, and they are identifiable as megakaryoblasts by their morphology or by other studies. These pleomorphic cells are often indistinguishable from other blasts on Romanowsky stains, but their true identity may be suspected when they have cytoplasmic projections or budding of platelets or when large, bizarre platelets or increased numbers of megakaryocytes are also present. Immunophenotypic studies, however, are necessary to confirm that the cells are genuinely megakaryoblasts. M7 constitutes about 2–4% of acute myeloid leukemias. This slide demonstrates one blast, which contains a large nucleus, one nucleolus, and scant basophilic cytoplasm from which rounded projections emanate. These projections suggest that the blast is in the megakaryocyte line, recapitulating the budding of platelets that normally occurs.

Acute Lymphoblastic Leukemia

According to the French-American-British (FAB) classification, the diagnosis of acute lymphoblastic leukemia (ALL) depends on demonstrating that at least 30% of the nucleated cells in a count of 500 bone marrow cells are lymphoblasts, when evaluated by special studies. The blasts in ALL are negative with histochemical stains that demonstrate cells of myeloid lineage—myeloperoxidase, Sudan black, and the esterases. Most ALL blasts show characteristic "blocks" of cytoplasmic PAS (periodic acid-Schiff). Immunophenotyping demonstrates that 75% of all cases of ALL have a B-cell lineage and about 25% are T-cells.

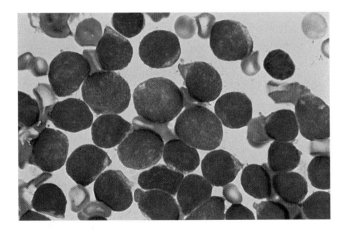

Slide 133. Acute Lymphoblastic Leukemia: Bone Marrow Aspirate

The predominant cell is small, possesses a regular nucleus with fairly homogeneous chromatin, and has a high nuclear:cytoplasm ratio. Nucleoli are absent or inconspicuous. Most cases of ALL have cells of this type. This aspirate demonstrates cells of fairly uniform size, containing very fine nuclear chromatin, absent nucleoli, and sparse cytoplasm.

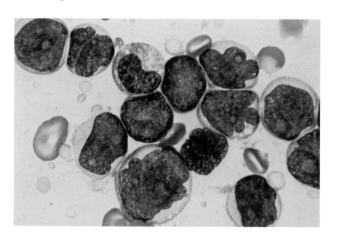

Slide 134. Acute Lymphoblastic Leukemia: Bone Marrow Aspirate

In some cases of acute lymphoblastic leukemia the blasts are larger and more variable, commonly have prominent nucleoli, and possess more abundant, often vacuolated, cytoplasm. The nuclei are irregular in outline and may be indented, folded, or cleft. Compared to the previous slide, the cells in this bone marrow aspirate are more pleomorphic, with coarser nuclear chromatin and greater irregularity in nuclear shape. In some cells, the cytoplasm is more substantial. Prominent nucleoli are present.

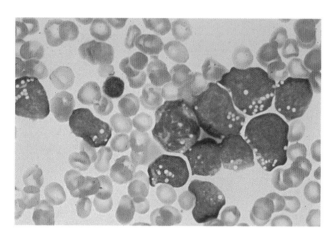

Slide 135. Lymphoma with Cells in the Peripheral Blood

Sometimes, the malignant cells of lymphomas may appear in large numbers within the peripheral circulation. These cases resemble acute lymphoblastic leukemia. Typically, the cells are large, and their cytoplasm is basophilic and commonly vacuolated. The regular-shaped, round, or oval nuclei may contain one or more nucleoli and uniform, dense, and finely-stippled chromatin. Vacuoles can occur in the nucleus, as demonstrated in this aspirate.

CHRONIC LYMPHOCYTIC LEUKEMIA

Chronic lymphocytic leukemia is a malignant disorder in which the primary problem is not an excessive production of abnormal lymphocytes but a protracted life span, causing their progressive accumulation. The cause is a defect in the steps that lead to programmed death, or apoptosis. In >95% of cases the leukemic lymphocyte is a B-cell. This disorder, the most common cause of leukemia in the United States, accounting for 25–30% of all cases, is primarily a disease of older adults, with the median age at diagnosis being about 55. Many patients are asymptomatic at presentation, the disease being discovered on routine blood tests. When symptoms develop, the most common are weakness, fatigue, and weight loss. In patients with hypogammaglobulinemia, frequent or severe bacterial infections may occur. The physical examination is often normal, but the commonest finding is enlargement of the cervical, axillary, and inguinal lymph nodes, which are firm, nontender, and movable. Hepatomegaly and splenomegaly, varying from mild to massive, may develop.

The diagnostic criteria for CLL are (1) an absolute blood lymphocytosis >5 × 10^9/L (5,000/mm³), with morphologically mature cells and lasting more than 4 weeks; (2) at least 30% lymphocytes in a normocellular or hypercellular marrow; and (3) a monoclonal B-cell phenotype of the predominant lymphocytes, with low levels of surface immunoglobulins and CD5 positivity. The lymphocytes appear mature on peripheral blood smear, but disrupted cells ("smudge cells") are common, indicating increased fragility, with damage to the cells occurring during preparation of the slide. Some patients have anemia, either from decreased production (because excessive lymphocytes in the bone marrow impair erythropoiesis) or from an autoimmune hemolytic anemia that occurs in 10–25% of patients sometime during their disease. The antibody is usually a warm-reactive, polyclonal IgG. Rarely, an immune-related red cell aplasia occurs. Thrombocytopenia can also develop from marrow suppression or, uncommonly, from an immune mechanism. Various staging systems exist that provide prognostic information. Patients with only lymphocytosis have a lengthy period of survival. When lymph node enlargement or hepatosplenomegaly accompanies the lymphocytosis, the prognosis is intermediate. Those with anemia or thrombocytopenia have the worst outcome. Other laboratory findings associated with a poor prognosis include increased serum LDH levels, hypoalbuminemia, and hypercalcemia.

Late complications of CLL include bacterial, viral, or fungal infections related to hypogammaglobulinemia, diminishing cell-mediated immunity, or neutropenia from the disease or its treatment. In about 1–10% of cases the disorder transforms into a non-Hodgkin's lymphoma (Richter's syndrome), usually of the large-cell variety, often developing suddenly with fever or other systemic symptoms and enlarging lymph nodes. In about 10% of patients with CLL, the disease transforms into prolymphocytic leukemia, with the lymphocyte changing to a large cell with nucleoli, convoluted nuclei, and immature chromatin. Rarely, patients develop paraneoplastic pemphigus, with blistering and ulceration of the skin and mucous membranes.

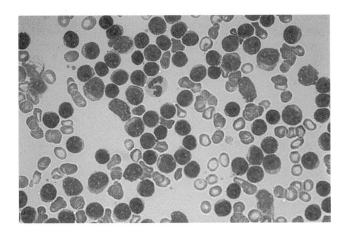

Slide 136. Chronic Lymphocytic Leukemia

In CLL, the lymphocytes usually appear normal, but they may be large or have deeply cleft nuclei (Reider cells). They sometimes contain coarse, clumped chromatin, and the cytoplasm may be vacuolated. With preparation of the blood film, lymphocytes commonly disintegrate. In these *smear* or *smudge* cells, the cytoplasm is lost and the nucleus spreads out.

Some of the cells may be prolymphocytes, which are larger than lymphocytes, have more abundant cytoplasm, possess a prominent nucleolus, and have a more condensed chromatin. Cases of CLL in which the prolymphocytes constitute 10–55% of the lymphoid cells are called CLL/PL. In others, lymphoid cells may vary from small to large, but prolymphocytes are less than 10%. These two variants of CLL are called chronic lymphocytic leukemia, mixed cell types. When prolymphocytes exceed 55% of the lymphoid cells, the disorder is called prolymphocytic leukemia (see slide 138).

When autoimmune hemolytic anemia complicates CLL, polychromatophilia and spherocytosis appear on the smear. Autoimmune thrombocytopenia may also occur. In this slide, lymphocytes, which constitute all the white cells except for one neutrophil, are fairly uniform in size and shape; a few smudge cells are scattered throughout the slide.

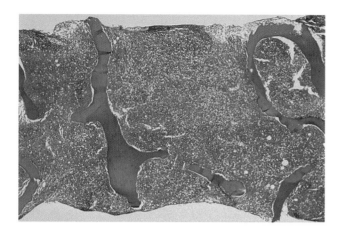

Slide 137. Chronic Lymphocytic Leukemia: Bone Marrow Biopsy

Patterns of bone marrow involvement include interstitial, nodular, diffuse, and mixed, which is a combination of nodular and interstitial. The type of pattern present has some prognostic significance, with the diffuse type having the most aggressive course. Nodular infiltrates are closely packed aggregates of cells that are usually not paratrabecular in location. In the interstitial pattern the lymphocytes intermingle with hematopoietic cells. In this slide, the bone marrow biopsy demonstrates the diffuse pattern.

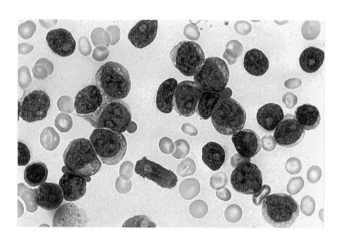

Slide 138. B-Cell Prolymphocytic Leukemia

When neoplastic prolymphocytes account for >55% of the lymphoid cells, the disorder is called prolymphocytic leukemia. T- and B-cell prolymphocytic leukemias are separate disorders. In the B-cell type the cells are larger than the lymphocytes in CLL, their nuclei have prominent nucleoli, and sometimes the cytoplasm is more abundant. The chromatin is moderately condensed. In the T-cell variety, the cells are more pleomorphic; the nuclear shape is irregular, often knobby; nucleoli are less prominent; the cytoplasm is scanty; and blebs may protrude from it. This slide reveals the characteristic appearance of prolymphocytes. In some, the cytoplasm is absent, and nucleoli are very prominent. In many cases this disorder may be an accelerated form of CLL, which often precedes it.

OTHER LEUKEMIAS

Hairy Cell Leukemia

Hairy cell leukemia accounts for about 2% of adult leukemias, with a male-female ratio of about 4:1 and an average age at diagnosis of approximately 50–55 years. The major clinical findings arise from infiltration of the bone marrow and spleen by a distinctive B-lymphocyte, the "hairy cell," causing pancytopenia and splenomegaly. The clinical features of pancytopenia include fatigue and other complaints related to anemia; easy bruising, petechiae, and ecchymoses from decreased platelets; and infections because of neutropenia, typically from gram-positive or gram-negative bacteria. Patients with hairy cell leukemia, however, also have an especial increased susceptibility to nontuberculous mycobacteria and fungi. *Toxoplasma gondii*, *Pneumocystis carinii*, *Listeria monocytogenes*, and various viruses may also cause infections, suggesting a diminished cell-mediated immunity. Indeed, nearly all patients have decreased numbers of monocytes. Palpable splenomegaly, sometimes to enormous dimensions, occurs in about 80–90% of patients. The liver is enlarged in approximately 30–40%. Hairy cell leukemia is the most common cause of paraneoplastic vasculitis, characterized by arthritis, palpable purpura, nodular skin lesions, and fever.

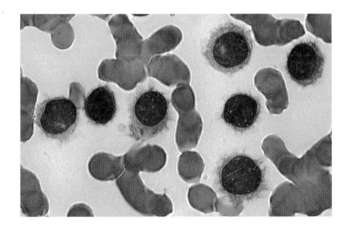

Slide 139. Hairy Cell Leukemia

Most patients have pancytopenia at presentation. Hairy cells are present in about 85% of peripheral smears. Larger than most other lymphocytes, with a diameter of 10–20 μm, these mononuclear cells have a round, oval, reniform, or dumbbell shape. The nucleus is often eccentric, round, or oval and contains diffuse chromatin. Nucleoli, when present, are small and inconspicuous. The abundant pale blue-gray and agranular cytoplasm has an uneven border with numerous irregular thin projections resembling hairs. This slide is taken from a thick part of the smear, accounting for the rouleaux, but white cells are often most abundant in these areas. All the cells are hairy cells, with easily visible cytoplasmic projections. Notice the diffuse chromatin in the nuclei and the gray-blue cytoplasm.

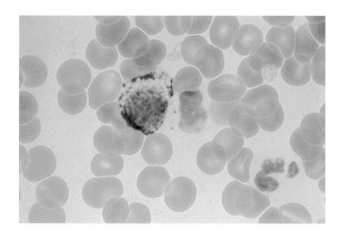

Slide 140. Hairy Cell Leukemia: TRAP Stain

Acid phosphatase activity is present in several types of blood cells. One form is an acid phosphatase resistant to tartrate. A tartrate-resistant acid phosphatase (TRAP) stain is positive in >95% of cases of hairy cell leukemia. Flow cytometric testing for surface markers specific for hairy cell leukemia, however, has replaced the TRAP stain as the preferred diagnostic test. In this slide, the hairy cell shows the red color that defines a positive TRAP reaction, which is absent from the two other myeloid cells. Cells are occasionally TRAP-positive in other disorders, such as infectious mononucleosis and chronic lymphocytic leukemia.

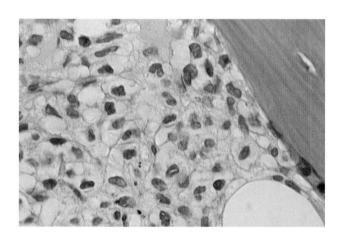

Slide 141. Hairy Cell Leukemia: Bone Marrow Biopsy

Bone marrow aspiration is frequently difficult or impossible in hairy cell leukemia because of associated fibrosis. On the biopsy, involvement by malignant cells may be patchy, focal, or diffuse. The abundant cytoplasm creates a substantial space between the nuclei of adjacent hairy cells, producing an appearance that resembles fried eggs. The nuclei, which demonstrate low mitotic activity, are round to oval and may be indented or bilobed. Reticulin fibrosis occurs in the areas of the hairy cells, its extent being proportional to the number of malignant cells present. In some cases the normal hematopoietic cells, especially granulocytic precursors, are markedly reduced, occasionally to the point of resembling aplastic anemia. A careful search for the hairy cells is then necessary to establish the proper diagnosis. This slide demonstrates infiltration of the hairy cells in the paratrabecular area. These are benign-appearing lymphoid cells with uniformly spaced nuclei because of the substantial cytoplasm characteristic of hairy cells.

Sézary's Syndrome

In 1938 Sézary and Bouvrain described a syndrome of pruritus, erythroderma, and hyperconvoluted lymphoid cells in the peripheral blood. This disorder, now considered a subset of cutaneous T-cell lymphoma, has an average age at onset of 55 and a male-female ratio of 2:1. Sézary's syndrome may be the initial manifestation of this malignant disorder or, more commonly, it develops in a patient with preceding cutaneous abnormalities of mycosis fungoides. These include scaly, erythematous macules and patches (the "eczematous" stage); sharply demarcated, scaly, and indurated erythematous to violaceous, elevated lesions (the "plaque" stage); or nodules and masses (the "tumor" stage). When Sézary's syndrome occurs, the skin becomes diffusely red and scaly, sometimes with infiltration and elevation of the facial structures ("leonine facies"), including the eyebrows, cheeks, and forehead. Palmar and plantar hyperkeratosis, hair loss, and abnormal fingernails are other dermatologic features. Constitutional findings include fever, chills, and weight loss. Sézary cells, which are activated T-cells, have hyperchromic and convoluted nuclei. They are present in varying numbers in Sézary's syndrome, their population often changing dramatically over short periods of time and their enumeration differing considerably among observers. Their presence signifies a poor prognosis. These cells, however, may also occur in cutaneous T-cell lymphomas in the absence of erythroderma and in benign skin diseases, including eczemas and the phenytoin hypersensitivity syndrome.

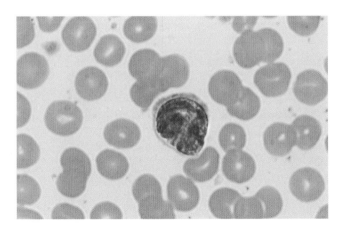

Slide 142. Sézary's Syndrome

In Sézary's syndrome the cells have a high nuclear: cytoplasm ratio and may be small (8–10 μm in diameter) or large (15–20 μm). The nuclei are convoluted, resembling the surface of a brain ("cerebriform"), and have dense chromatin. Nucleoli are commonly absent or inconspicuous, but may be visible in the large-cell variety. The cytoplasm is typically basophilic, agranular, and often vacuolated. The lymphoid cell in this slide is big, has scanty cytoplasm, and contains a large cleft, cerebriform nucleus.

LYMPHOMAS

The lymphomas constitute a heterogeneous group of neoplastic lymphocytic disorders, usually arising from lymph nodes. Less commonly they originate in other tissues, including the bone marrow, gut, spleen, liver, and skin. They are classified as either Hodgkin's disease or non-Hodgkin's lymphoma (NHL), the latter further divided into B-cell and T-cell types. Bone marrow examination is commonly part of the initial staging of lymphoma and is valuable in assessing the response to treatment, including chemotherapy, radiation, or bone marrow transplantation. Marrow involvement by lymphoma is usually from disseminated disease, but a significant discrepancy often exists between the morphology seen in the lymph nodes and that in trephine marrow biopsies. For this reason, accurate classification of lymphomas solely by the bone marrow findings is usually not possible. With marrow involvement, the lymphoma is best detected by generous bilateral iliac crest trephine biopsies, but other samples to evaluate include touch imprints, aspirate smears, clot sections, and peripheral blood smears. Aspirated material permits additional studies, including immunophenotyping, cytogenetics, and molecular assays. Manual disaggregation of fresh trephine biopsies into tissue culture media also provides specimens for ancillary tests such as flow cytometry and cytogenetics.

Bone marrow involvement by lymphoma is common. Over 80% of patients with low-grade variants of B-cell NHL have lymphoma in the marrow at the time of presentation. The standard method to evaluate bone marrow from patients with lymphoma is to examine thin-cut, H&E-stained specimens from formalin-fixed, paraffin-embedded core biopsy specimens. Biopsies are best viewed at low-power magnification to discern focal disruptions of overall architecture, such as aggregates primarily comprising lymphoid cells or abnormal collections of inflammatory cells (lymphocytes, plasma cells, histiocytes, and eosinophils). Other abnormal architectural patterns detected at low power include many manifestations of Hodgkin's disease, namely, foci of necrosis, fibrosis, or granulomatous inflammation.

Bone marrow involvement by NHL typically consists of a diffuse effacement of normal marrow architecture or of discrete, neoplastic lymphoid aggregates. Compared to the benign aggregates described below, the neoplastic ones are more numerous, larger, and composed entirely of monotonous, medium to large lymphoid cells with irregular nuclear contours. Lymphoid aggregates that reside exclusively in paratrabecular locations indicate marrow involvement by follicular center–derived B-cell NHL. If the morphological findings are suspicious on H&E stains, flow cytometry can often readily confirm bone marrow involvement by demonstrating abnormal lymphoma-specific immunophenotypes (such as surface light chain restriction in B-cell NHL).

Benign lymphoid aggregates are common in marrow biopsy sections. They are more frequent in the elderly and are often associated with other disorders, such as infections, autoimmune diseases, and myeloproliferative syndromes. Benign lymphoid aggregates are usually small, well-circumscribed aggregates consisting of a moderately pleomorphic population of small, regular lymphocytes admixed with other inflammatory cells, including macrophages and plasma cells. They are often found near small blood vessels and virtually never in paratrabecular locations.

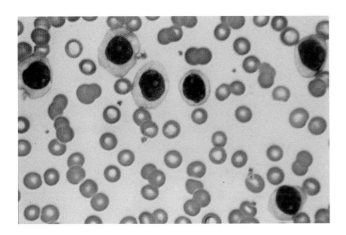

Slide 143. Non-Hodgkin's Lymphoma: Peripheral Blood

Sometimes lymphoma cells are visible on peripheral smears in low numbers. This finding is usually seen in one of two clinical settings: (1) primary involvement of the bone marrow or spleen by a chronic lymphoproliferative disorder, or (2) secondary involvement of blood from disseminated node- or extranodal-based NHL. The former includes CLL, prolymphocytic lymphoma, hairy cell leukemia, and large granular lymphocytic leukemia. This blood smear, an unusual example of peripheral lymphocytosis (or "leukemic phase") attributable to numerous circulating marginal zone B-cell lymphoma cells, contains six atypical lymphoid cells with monocytoid features.

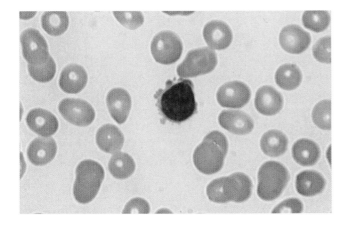

Slide 144. Splenic Lymphoma with Villous Lymphocytes: Peripheral Blood

This indolent, low-grade B-cell lymphoma characteristically occurs in elderly men, who have splenomegaly, little or no lymph node enlargement, mild anemia and thrombocytopenia, and a moderate leukocytosis composed of atypical lymphocytes. These cells are slightly larger than normal small lymphocytes and have a round or oval nucleus with condensed chromatin and, often, a nucleolus. The cytoplasm is sparse to moderate and basophilic, with villous projections that are often bipolar—that is, occurring at two sites 180 degrees apart. Plasmacytoid lymphocytes may also occur. Most patients have positive marrow samples, with focal involvement more frequent than diffuse. This peripheral blood smear demonstrates a lymphocyte with a slightly oval nucleus, moderately condensed chromatin, and numerous, somewhat bulbous projections from the gray-blue cytoplasm.

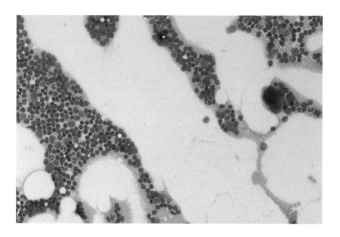

Slide 145. Non-Hodgkin's Lymphoma: Bone Marrow Aspirate

This slide is a medium-power view of an aspirate that shows a proliferation of small and medium-sized mononuclear cells with high nuclear:cytoplasmic ratios and round, regular nuclei with closed chromatin. These abnormal lymphoid cells constitute the majority of the marrow cells in this field. A megakaryocyte is seen on the right, but most of the erythroid and myeloid series are markedly reduced in number. This patient suffered from large-cell non-Hodgkin's lymphoma.

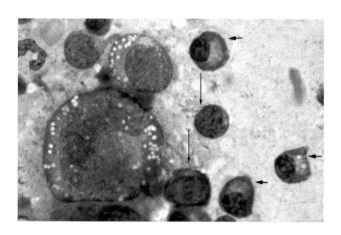

Slide 146. Non-Hodgkin's Lymphoma: Bone Marrow Aspirate

Non-Hodgkin's lymphoma is a morphologically heterogeneous group of disorders that often include cellular components with both benign and malignant appearances. Because aspirate smears may not represent the bone marrow cavity as a whole, morphological interpretation to assess marrow involvement by lymphoma is best done in conjunction with biopsy interpretation. Often histochemical and immunophenotypical analysis, in addition to routine Romanowsky stains, are necessary to evaluate these cases. This slide, from an anaplastic large-cell lymphoma (an aggressive T-cell lymphoma), shows a very large malignant cell with irregular nuclear borders, multiple large nucleoli, and vacuolated basophilic cytoplasm. Accompanying this large bizarre cell is another malignant vacuolated lymphoma cell, and to the right are three plasma cells (*short horizontal arrows*) and two atypical lymphocytes (*long vertical arrows*).

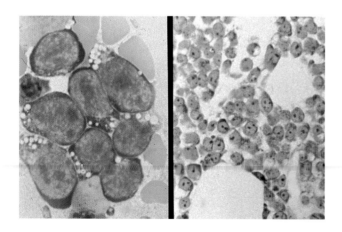

Slide 147. Burkitt's Lymphoma: Bone Marrow Aspirate and Biopsy

Burkitt's lymphoma is an aggressive B-cell lymphoproliferative disorder that usually arises in extranodal sites. In adults, the nonendemic variety predominates and most often presents with abdominal pain and swelling. The left side of this composite slide shows an aspirate smear with eight Burkitt lymphoma cells having characteristic morphology: an open chromatin pattern with several prominent nucleoli and ample vacuolated, immature, blue cytoplasm. On the right side of the slide is the corresponding biopsy specimen showing monotonous sheets of atypical lymphoid cells with conspicuous nucleoli and ample basophilic, vacuolated cytoplasm.

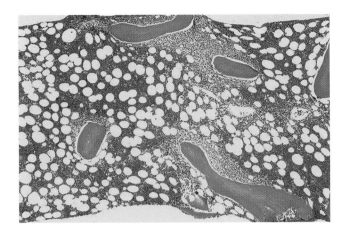

Slide 148. Non-Hodgkin's Lymphoma: Biopsy

Non-Hodgkin's lymphoma involves the bone marrow in approximately one-third to one-half of patients at the time of diagnosis. Microscopic patterns of involvement can be focal, interstitial, or diffuse, and, depending on the type of lymphoma, may have prognostic significance. This slide shows a paratrabecular pattern typical of non-Hodgkin's lymphoma arising from follicular center B-cells, in which the malignant lymphocytes disrupt marrow architecture by forming discrete nodules around bony trabeculae.

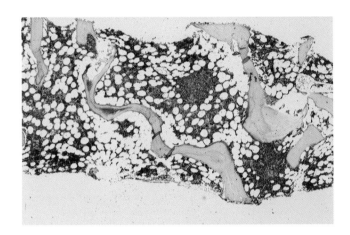

Slide 149. Non-Hodgkin's Lymphoma: Bone Marrow Biopsy

Bone marrow involvement by non-Hodgkin's lymphoma is usually apparent as either discrete atypical lymphoid aggregates or as effacement with a diffuse increase in atypical lymphoid cells. The cellular composition is highly variable and may not even represent the cell type seen in the lymph nodes from which the lymphoma originated. The bone marrow lymphomatous nodule may be composed entirely of a monotonous lymphoid cell or may include other inflammatory cells such as eosinophils, macrophages, and plasma cells. Compared to normal benign lymphoid aggregates (see slide 84), lymphomatous nodules are usually numerous, large, poorly circumscribed, and, in follicular center–derived B-cell varieties, paratrabecular in location. This slide, from a patient with diffuse large-cell non-Hodgkin's lymphoma, is an example of nodular involvement in the marrow, showing three lymphomatous nodules, two paratrabecular and one midtrabecular in location.

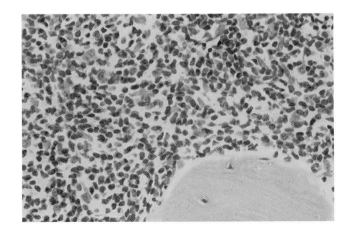

Slide 150. Non-Hodgkin's Lymphoma: Bone Marrow Biopsy

Non-Hodgkin's lymphomas constitute a diverse spectrum of diseases. They are neoplastic proliferations of both B- and T-cells with quite varied morphological features on microscopic examination, ranging from heterogeneous collections of benign hematopoietic cells that accompany many of the T-cell lymphomas to a monotonous proliferation of highly atypical large lymphoid cells characteristic of the large B-cell lymphomas. This slide from a biopsy specimen shows numerous large atypical lymphoid cells in a paratrabecular location.

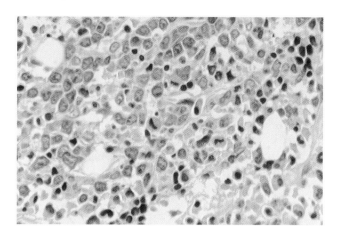

Slide 151. Non-Hodgkin's Lymphoma: Bone Marrow Biopsy

This high-power view of a biopsy specimen from a patient with diffuse large-cell non-Hodgkin's lymphoma shows prominent numbers of highly atypical large lymphoid cells with vesicular (or "bubbly") chromatin and one or two nucleoli. These large lymphoma cells have highly irregular nuclear contours with an overall highly pleomorphic appearance—all features of a malignant cell. In the background, small lymphocytes are scattered diffusely throughout.

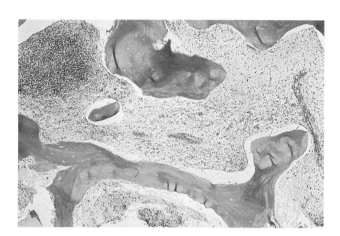

Slide 152. Hodgkin's Lymphoma: Bone Marrow Biopsy

Hodgkin's lymphoma involves the marrow in about 10% of cases at the time of the initial diagnosis. The morphological appearance is most often of a fibrotic process accompanied by a reactive collection of different inflammatory cells, including small and large lymphocytes, histiocytes, eosinophils, and plasma cells. The diagnostic malignant cell of Hodgkin's lymphoma, the Reed-Sternberg cell, is often present, but more commonly atypical large histiocytic cells predominate. The Reed-Sternberg cell is a large multinucleated cell containing inclusion-like, pink nucleoli with abundant clear cytoplasm. Because of the large amount of fibrosis present, attempts at bone marrow aspiration are often unsuccessful (dry taps). This slide is a low-power view showing disruption of normal marrow architecture by an obliterative fibrotic process with a single hypercellular focus in the upper left portion of the slide composed primarily of small lymphocytes. The bony trabeculae are thickened, a common reaction associated with fibrosis.

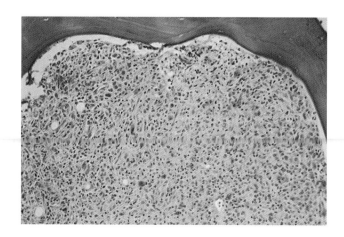

Slide 153. Hodgkin's Disease: Bone Marrow Biopsy

This hypercellular biopsy demonstrates a mixture of inflammatory cells and spindle-shaped fibroblasts. The inflammatory cells include small lymphocytes with slightly irregular dark-staining nuclei, plasma cells, eosinophils, and larger atypical cells with open vesicular nuclei—atypical Reed-Sternberg cells.

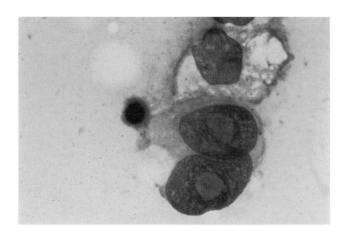

Slide 154. Hodgkin's Disease: Bone Marrow Aspirate

This slide from a case of Hodgkin's lymphoma involving the marrow demonstrates a diagnostic binucleate Reed-Sternberg cell with characteristic inclusion-type nucleoli and clear-staining cytoplasm, an unusual finding in aspirates.

PLASMA CELL DISORDERS

Multiple Myeloma

Multiple myeloma is a malignancy of plasma cells of unknown cause, although radiation exposure is a predisposing factor in some patients. The median age at diagnosis is about 65, and it is about twice as common in blacks as whites. Its clinical manifestations arise from (1) the presence of numerous malignant plasma cells, usually in the bone marrow; (2) the effects of a monoclonal protein in the blood or urine produced by the malignant cells; or (3) the immunologic deficiencies caused when the immunoglobulin production by remaining normal plasma cells is inadequate.

This disorder commonly causes several bone lesions, which gave rise to its name, multiple myeloma (tumor of the bone marrow). Some patients, however, have only a single lesion, and others have diffuse osteopenia, rather than discrete areas of osteolysis, because of the widespread presence of malignant cells throughout the bones. These skeletal abnormalities develop because the malignant cells produce substances that cause bone absorption and impair bone formation. One clinical manifestation is bone pain, which can occur from vertebral compression fractures or from osteolytic lesions in other sites. On radiographs, these lytic areas often have a sharp margin, especially in the skull and long bones. In the pelvis, ribs, and vertebrae, their radiologic appearance may be more mottled and indistinct. Another complication of bone involvement is hypercalcemia, causing lethargy, confusion, and constipation. In addition, the presence of polyuria, nausea, and vomiting from the increased calcium can lead to intravascular volume depletion and renal failure. In about two-thirds of patients, the presence of malignant plasma cells in the bone marrow impairs erythropoiesis, causing anemia.

Tumors of plasma cells can also form outside the marrow (extramedullary plasmacytoma), presenting as masses in the skin, lymph nodes, liver, spleen, and other locations. They may be solitary and unassociated with any other evidence of multiple myeloma.

In nearly all patients the myeloma cells produce an abnormal monoclonal (M) protein, which is IgG in about 60%, IgA in 20%, and light chains only (κ in about two-thirds; λ in about one-third) in 20%. Immunoelectrophoresis and immunofixation of blood and urine reveals an M protein in 99% of patients. A serious complication of this protein is renal failure, typically caused by the formation in the renal tubules of casts consisting of immunoglobulin and free light chains (Bence Jones protein), which about 80% of patients with multiple myeloma excrete in the urine. M proteins can also cause glomerular damage in some patients. In fewer than 10% of patients these paraproteins, usually IgA, form enough polymers to cause hyperviscosity, producing decreased visual acuity, bleeding, and neurologic manifestations such as dizziness, headache, confusion, vertigo, and ataxia. Excess light chains may result in AL amyloidosis, present in as many as 35% of patients with multiple myeloma and usually manifested by the carpal tunnel syndrome and proteinuria. In the absence of amyloid, a symmetrical sensorimotor peripheral neuropathy can develop from the toxic effect of some paraproteins on peripheral nerves. This complication particularly occurs in a syndrome that can include hepatosplenomegaly, lymph node enlargement, diabetes mellitus, erectile dysfunction, gynecomastia, diffuse cutaneous hyperpigmentation, and lesions in the bones that are sclerotic rather than lytic. This disorder is called osteosclerotic myeloma, Crow-Fukase syndrome, or POEMS, an acronym for *p*olyneuropathy, *o*rganomegaly, *e*ndocrinopathy, *M*-protein, and *s*kin changes.

A diminution in normal immunoglobulin production can cause an increased susceptibility to infections, especially from two bacteria with polysaccharide capsules, *Streptococcus pneumoniae* and *Hemophilus influenzae*. Infections with gram-negative bacilli are also common, sometimes arising from neutropenia caused by disease progression or chemotherapy.

In one scheme, the diagnosis of multiple myeloma depends on the presence of one major and one minor criteria or three minor criteria. The major criteria are (1) plasmacytoma on tissue biopsy; (2) plasma cells constituting at least 30% of the marrow cells; (3) a monoclonal serum protein (IgG > 3.5 g/dL; IgA > 2 g/dL); or urine secretion of Bence Jones protein of at least 1 g/24 hours. The minor criteria are (1) marrow plasmacytosis of 10–29%; (2) monoclonal proteins present in less than the quantity specified in the major criteria; (3) lytic bone lesions; (4) decreased uninvolved immunoglobulins (IgM < 50 mg/dL; IgA < 100 mg/dL; IgG < 600 mg/dL).

Because the plasma cells in multiple myeloma produce increased immunoglobulin (paraprotein), which is acidic and takes up the basophilic stain, the background color on slides of peripheral blood may be bluer than usual. The paraprotein causes red cells to adhere, and the resulting rouleaux may be visible on those portions of the smear where erythrocytes are normally separated. Anemia is usual, and the red cells are ordinarily normochromic and normocytic, but occasionally macrocytic. Leukoerythroblastosis, the presence of nucleated erythrocytes and immature granulocytes, is sometimes present. A few plasmacytoid lymphocytes and plasma cells are often detectable. The bone marrow characteristically discloses increased plasma cells, which may appear cytologically normal or have features of altered maturation, such as a high nuclear:cytoplasmic ratio, nucleoli, a diffuse nuclear chromatin pattern, bilobed nuclei, and mitoses. Some plasma cells can have peripheral cytoplasmic eosinophilia (flame cells). Inclusions in the plasma cells represent increased immunoglobulin synthesis: large, homogeneous hyaline material called Russell bodies when in the cytoplasm and Dutcher bodies when in the nucleus. Plasma cells containing numerous inclusions are called Mott, grape, or morular cells. None of these findings is specific for multiple myeloma; all may be present in benign plasmacytosis.

On biopsy, the patterns of involvement are interstitial, with the myeloma cells interspersed with the normal hematopoietic cells; nodular, in which masses of cells usually occur away from the paratrabecular areas; and diffuse or "packed" marrow, with solid areas in which the plasma cells replace fat and normal hematopoietic components.

Plasma cell leukemia is arbitrarily defined as an absolute plasma cell count in the blood of $>2{,}000/\text{mm}^3$ ($2 \times 10^9/\text{L}$) associated with a neoplastic proliferation of monoclonal plasma cells. It occurs in about 1–4% of cases of multiple myeloma, either as the presenting feature or as a transformation of a previously diagnosed case.

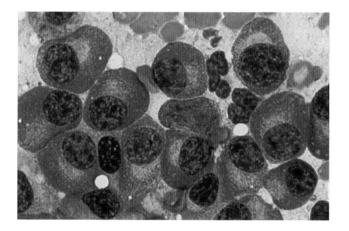

Slide 155. Multiple Myeloma: Bone Marrow Aspirate

On bone marrow aspirates, plasma cells are usually increased and may constitute nearly all the cells. Their appearance may be normal, but atypical features are often present, including large size, mitotic figures, multinuclearity, nuclear-cytoplasmic asynchrony in maturation, prominent nucleoli, phagocytosis of other cells by the plasma cells, and absence of the Golgi zone. In this slide, nearly all the cells are plasma cells.

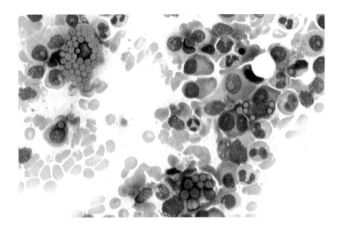

Slide 156. Multiple Myeloma: Bone Marrow Aspirate

In this slide, many of the nucleated cells are neoplastic plasma cells. Nucleoli are often prominent, and the Golgi zone varies from prominent to absent. Several are Mott cells with numerous cytoplasmic inclusions, and in one cell in the left upper corner, these inclusions obscure the cytoplasm altogether.

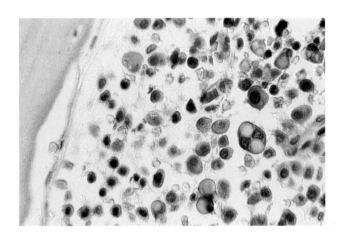

Slide 157. Multiple Myeloma: Bone Marrow Biopsy

This biopsy demonstrates a pleomorphic population of plasma cells. Several are Mott cells with intracytoplasmic inclusions. Note the characteristic eccentric nuclei in the plasma cells.

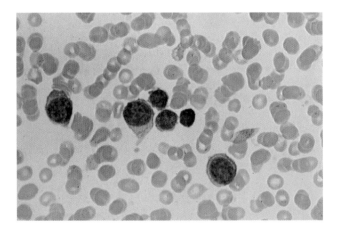

Slide 158. Plasma Cell Leukemia

In plasma cell leukemia, the circulating plasma cells may appear normal, but often have the atypical features described in slide 155. This blood smear discloses rouleaux. Several pleomorphic lymphoid cells are recognizable as plasma cells by the coarsely clumped nuclear chromatin, the eccentric nuclei, and the bluish-gray color of the cytoplasm. Chromatin may clump in several sites at the periphery of the nucleus, causing it to resemble the markings on a clock face. A spectrum of pleomorphic lymphoid cells is present, ranging from large, atypical plasmacytoid forms to normal small lymphocytes.

Waldenström's Macroglobulinemia

Waldenström's macroglobulinemia, which accounts for about 2% of adult hematologic malignancies, is a clonal disorder of B-cells in which excessive amounts of IgM are produced. It occurs almost exclusively in older adults, with a median age at diagnosis in the mid-60s and a slight male predominance. Constitutional clinical features of fatigue and weight loss are common. The main manifestations of the disease develop from (1) tissue infiltration by malignant B-cells, especially in the bone marrow, lymph nodes, and spleen; (2) the effects of excessive *circulating* IgM, including hyperviscosity, cryoglobulinemia, and cold-agglutinin anemia; and (3) the results of excessive *tissue* IgM. Neuropathy, glomerular disease, or amyloidosis can occur. Lymph node enlargement and splenomegaly are present in about 20–40% of patients. Unusual areas of tumor invasion include the lung, gastrointestinal tract, and skin.

Hyperviscosity causes several problems. Visual blurring and decreased acuity are accompanied by funduscopic findings of dilated and tortuous retinal veins, with segmented dilations ("sausage links" or "boxcars"), hemorrhages, exudates, and papilledema. Neurologic manifestations, probably from vascular sludging, include fatigue, dizziness, headache, deafness, tinnitus, nystagmus, confusion, vertigo, and ataxia. Bleeding, manifested by epistaxis, oral mucosal hemorrhage, or purpura, is frequent and arises from capillary damage due to hyperviscosity as well as from IgM interactions with platelets and coagulation factors. The plasma volume is commonly increased, sometimes leading to congestive heart failure and cerebral hemorrhages. Cryoglobulins may cause Raynaud's phenomenon, cold urticaria, arthralgias, purpura, peripheral neuropathy, renal failure, and vascular occlusion, while cold agglutinins can produce a hemolytic anemia.

Tissue deposition of IgM in nerves can cause a chronic, predominantly demyelinating sensorimotor peripheral neuropathy, which occurs in about 5–10% of patients. Glomerular deposition of IgM may lead to proteinuria, which is usually mild and reversible. Amyloidosis develops in less than 5% of patients, producing the nephrotic syndrome, renal failure, cardiac failure, and pulmonary involvement.

A normocytic, normochromic anemia is common and has several causes, including bone marrow infiltration, hemolysis, bleeding, and dilution from hyperviscosity-related increased plasma volume. On blood smear, rouleaux formation is typically present, red cell agglutination may occur, and erythrophagocytosis may be visible. Lymphocytes are often increased and may resemble plasma cells ("plasmacytoid lymphocytes").

IgM levels are typically >1g/dL. Other laboratory findings include an increased erythrocyte sedimentation rate, often exceeding 100 mm/hr; hyperuricemia; hyperviscosity, usually with IgM levels >3g/dL; hyponatremia; and hypercalcemia in about 4%.

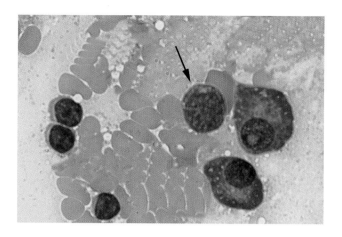

Slide 159. Waldenström's Macroglobulinemia: Bone Marrow Aspirate

As in multiple myeloma, the excessive amount of immunoglobulin may give an increased bluish color to the background and cause rouleaux formation on the peripheral blood smear. Because the paraprotein is IgM, substantial red cell agglutination may also occur. The erythrocytes are normochromic and normocytic. In many patients lymphocytes are increased; these appear normal or have plasmacytoid features. In this bone marrow aspirate, two atypical plasma cells are present; one, on the right, has a prominent nucleolus. A plasmacytoid lymphocyte (*arrow*) appears to the left of them. Three normal small lymphocytes lie on the left side.

Systemic Amyloidosis

Amyloidosis occurs from the extracellular deposition of homogeneous protein molecules that aggregate to form nonbranching fibrils that, when stained with Congo red, give an apple-green birefringence under polarized light. On electron microscopy, they have a β-pleated sheet pattern, thought to be responsible for the staining characteristics. Several amyloid types exist, each deriving from normal human protein precursors. Light chains, λ about 2–3 times as frequently as κ, can polymerize to form an amyloid called AL (amyloid, light-chain-related), which causes primary amyloidosis. Amyloid fibrils in secondary amyloidosis and in familial Mediterranean fever consist of amyloid A, which arises from portions of a circulating serum protein (SAA) produced by hepatocytes. Levels of SAA rise significantly with inflammation, and amyloid A is most commonly seen in chronic inflammatory conditions. Some systemic amyloidoses are hereditary, and the amyloid in them forms from abnormal types of transthyretin, a plasma protein that carries thyroxine and retinol-binding protein. Other precursor proteins in various amyloids include gelsolin, present in the cytoplasm; lysozyme, an antibacterial substance found in several body fluids; and β_2-microglobulin, a light chain on the surface of cells expressing MHC class 1 antigen that is catabolized by the proximal tubular cells and accumulates to cause amyloid in patients with chronic renal failure undergoing dialysis. The diagnosis of any of these disorders requires demonstration of amyloid in tissue and subsequently immunohistochemical staining to identify the specific type present.

The most common variety, primary amyloidosis (AL), occurs in males about twice as commonly as in females and is usually diagnosed at about age 60. Sometimes the origin of the light chains is multiple myeloma or Waldenström's macroglobulinemia. The most common symptoms are weakness, fatigue, and weight loss. The clinical manifestations depend on which organs contain amyloid; virtually any may be involved. Infiltration of the tongue can cause macroglossia. With renal deposition, proteinuria leading to hypoalbuminemia and peripheral edema is common. Renal failure may occur, sometimes abruptly. Amyloid deposition in the heart may cause conduction defects, arrhythmias, and congestive heart failure from a restrictive cardiomyopathy with normal systolic function but impaired diastolic filling. A symmetrical, predominantly sensory, peripheral neuropathy can occur, causing paresthesias and numbness, primarily in the lower extremities. Amyloid deposition in the carpal tunnel can compress the median nerve, leading to the carpal tunnel syndrome. Accumulation of amyloid in the autonomic nervous system can produce orthostatic hypotension, gastrointestinal motility disorders, impotence, abnormal sweating, and bladder dysfunction. Involvement of the liver causes hepatomegaly, sometimes with portal hypertension, and amyloid deposition in the spleen produces splenomegaly, sometimes leading to splenic rupture and hypofunction. With infiltration of the gastrointestinal tract, malabsorption, hemorrhage, protein loss, obstruction, and ulceration may occur. Cutaneous findings include nodules, tumors, and purpura, which arises from vascular fragility caused by amyloid infiltration of the vessel walls and impaired coagulation because factor X binds to amyloid. A common site of ecchymoses is periorbital.

Anemia, when present, is usually mild, but a blood smear may show signs of splenic hypofunction—thrombocytosis and Howell-Jolly bodies. Serum and urine electrophoresis and immunofixation identify a monoclonal protein in about 90–95% of patients. Bone marrow examination shows normal or mildly increased numbers of plasma cells, unless multiple myeloma is present. On bone marrow biopsy, amyloid deposits are detectable in about 50–60% of patients, either in the walls of small blood vessels or in extravascular spaces. They are homogeneous pink areas that demonstrate apple-green birefringence with polarized light after staining with Congo red. In most cases of AL amyloidosis, fine-needle subcutaneous fat aspirates of the abdominal wall or bone marrow biopsy can establish the diagnosis. If these are negative, biopsy of the rectal mucosa or of a clinically involved organ is appropriate.

In most systemic amyloidoses other than AL, the organs involved include the heart, kidney, and peripheral nervous system; the bone marrow is usually unaffected. Secondary amyloidosis is an exception. This disorder occurs in chronic inflammatory conditions, with amyloid formed from serum amyloid A (SAA), an acute-phase reactant that increases in inflammation. In the United States, the most common cause is rheumatoid arthritis, but other diseases seen in this country include osteomyelitis, bronchiectasis, inflammatory bowel disease, renal cell carcinoma, familial Mediterranean fever, and other rheumatic diseases, such as ankylosing spondylitis, psoriatic arthritis, and systemic lupus erythematosus. The organ most commonly involved is the kidney, causing proteinuria and renal insufficiency. The gastrointestinal tract is clinically affected in about 20%, with diarrhea, decreased motility, and malabsorption being the major manifestations. Sites where biopsies are commonly positive include thin-needle aspiration of subcutaneous abdominal fat, bone marrow (about 50%), rectum, kidney, stomach or small bowel, and liver.

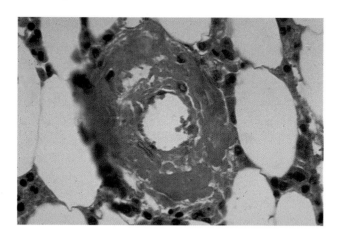

Slide 160. Light Chain (AL) Amyloidosis: Bone Marrow Biopsy

In AL amyloidosis, the peripheral blood smear may be unremarkable or may show rouleaux and enhanced background staining because of high immunoglobulin levels. The bone marrow cells may be normal, or plasma cells may be increased. In this bone marrow biopsy specimen, pink-staining material infiltrates the vessel wall; special stains demonstrated that it was amyloid.

Platelet Disorders

THROMBOTIC THROMBOCYTOPENIC PURPURA

In this disease, platelet thrombi form in the arterioles and capillaries throughout the body. No predisposing factors are usually apparent, but some medications such as ticlopidine and cyclosporine seem to cause it. Women are more frequently affected than men, and most patients are between 20 and 60 years of age. The pathogenesis appears to be related to the presence in the blood of large polymers of von Willebrand's factor, which is secreted by the vascular endothelial cells into the circulation. Ordinarily an enzyme breaks these substances down, but in thrombotic thrombocytopenic purpura this proteinase is absent or inactivated by an antibody. The large polymers that accumulate cause platelet clumping, which occludes the microvasculature and damages erythrocytes as they travel through the vessels.

Five major clinical features occur in this disease—fever, neurologic abnormalities, renal failure, thrombocytopenia, and microangiopathic hemolytic anemia; the last two are essential to the diagnosis. The most common findings at presentation are bleeding, usually cutaneous, in the form of petechiae or ecchymoses, but sometimes mucosal, such as epistaxis, melena, or hematochezia; fatigue (probably attributable to anemia); neurologic symptoms; and abdominal pain. The neurologic abnormalities are often multifocal and transient; these include headache, confusion, seizures, visual changes (usually from hemorrhage into the retina or vitreous), cranial nerve palsies, and focal findings such as aphasia and paresis. The source of the abdominal pain is uncertain, but it may arise from organ ischemia or hemorrhage. Renal manifestations consist of proteinuria, hematuria, casts, and usually mild elevations in serum creatinine and urea nitrogen levels. Acute, often oliguric, renal failure can occur. Heart failure, arrhythmias, and conduction abnormalities may develop, probably from myocardial ischemia due to thrombi in the coronary vessels.

The thrombocytopenia is usually profound, with platelet levels commonly less than 20,000/mm³. Anemia is present at presentation or develops shortly thereafter, but tends to be moderate, with hematocrits usually in the 20s. The white cell count is commonly increased. The LDH level is markedly elevated from hemolysis and tissue ischemia. Indirect bilirubin rises and the haptoglobin level diminishes because of the intravascular hemolysis. Hemosiderin and hemoglobin may be present in the urine.

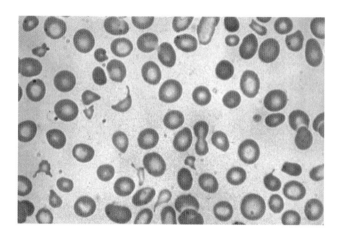

Slide 161. Thrombotic Thrombocytopenic Purpura

In this disease, the characteristic findings on the peripheral blood smear include a severe decrease in platelets, impressive polychromasia (often accompanied by nucleated red cells), and schistocytes, which are irregularly shaped erythrocyte fragments. Bone marrow samples demonstrate hyperplasia of megakaryocytes and red cell precursors. In biopsies, platelet thrombi may be visible in the arterioles. In this peripheral smear, platelets are decreased, and several fragmented erythrocytes are present throughout the field, including helmet cells and microspherocytes.

Infections

BACTERIA

To be visible on a regular peripheral blood smear, bacteria must reach a density of about 10^5 organisms/mL of blood. Even if a slide is made from a buffy coat (a concentrated preparation of white cells and platelets made after centrifugation of blood), bacteria are generally detectable only when their numbers exceed about 10^4/mL of blood. This intensity of bacteremia rarely occurs: in most patients with positive blood cultures, <500 bacteria/mL are present. Occasionally, however, when overwhelming sepsis develops, organisms are visible on a regular peripheral blood smear. Many different types have been seen, including *Staphylococcus aureus*, *Neisseria meningitidis*, *Streptococcus pneumoniae*, and various gram-negative bacilli.

Such high-level bacteremia can occur in asplenic hosts infected with *Streptococcus pneumoniae*, a gram-positive diplococcus. Since both this organism and the gram-negative diplococcus, *Neisseria meningitidis*, stain blue with Romanowsky dyes, they can be differentiated on the Wright stain only by their shape and size. Pneumococci are oval and lie end-to-end; meningococci are larger, appear kidney-shaped, and lie side-by-side. A Gram stain of the smear can determine whether the organism is gram-positive or gram-negative.

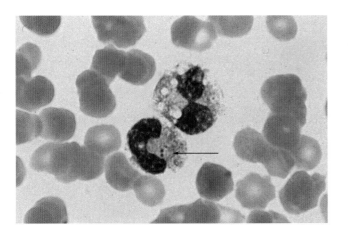

Slide 162. Pneumococcal Bacteremia

A pair of oval-shaped organisms lying end-to-end (*arrow*) is visible in the cytoplasm of the lower white cell (a band) in this asplenic patient with bacteremia from *Streptococcus pneumoniae*. The upper granulocyte shows extensive cytoplasmic vacuolization, a finding often present in severe infections.

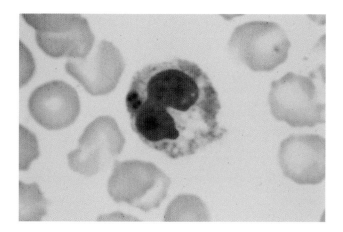

Slide 163. Meningococcal Bacteremia

Two pairs of bacteria lie in the cytoplasm of this neutrophil, which also has vacuoles. Each set of organisms consists of two kidney-shaped bacteria lying side-by-side. Blood cultures yielded *Neisseria meningitidis*.

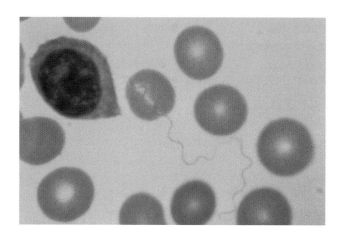

Slide 164. Borreliosis (Relapsing Fever)

Relapsing fever is an infection by certain *Borrelia* species that consists of recurrent episodes of chills, fever, headache, and fatigue lasting a few days, followed by a few days of apyrexia. During the febrile episodes the *Borrelia* spirochetes causing this disease are usually visible on routine blood smears, which is the best procedure in establishing the diagnosis. The organisms are 7–20 μm long and about 0.7 μm in diameter. *Borrelia recurrentis*, which has no animal reservoir, is spread from person to person by body lice and exists in Africa, China, and the Peruvian Andes. Tickborne disease, whose major reservoirs are wild rodents, occurs in the western United States as well as many other countries throughout the world and is caused by several different *Borrelia* species. In this slide, two contiguous threadlike spiral organisms are visible.

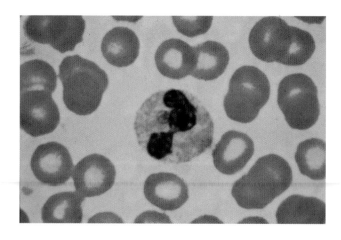

Slide 165. Ehrlichiosis

The genus *Ehrlichia* consists of obligate intracellular gram-negative bacteria that can be transmitted by ticks to humans from their mammalian hosts, which include horses, deer, and dogs. On Romanowsky stains of the peripheral blood, these organisms may be visible inside the cytoplasm of granulocytes or monocytes, depending on the species of *Ehrlichia*. They appear, often in vacuoles, as dark blue bacteria in loose or dense aggregates called morulae because of their resemblance to mulberries. Infection with these organisms causes fever, headache, myalgias, increased liver enzymes, and progressive pancytopenia. In this patient with granulocytic ehrlichiosis, a morula is present just to the left of the central lobe of this neutrophil.

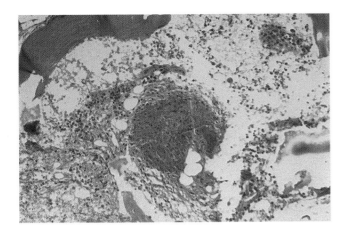

Slide 166. Mycobacteria: Bone Marrow Biopsy

Disseminated infection with various *Mycobacterium* species, including *M. tuberculosis*, typically causes fever and anemia, but other cytopenias, leukemoid reactions (marked increase in neutrophils), monocytosis, thrombocytosis, and leukoerythroblastosis may also occur. Bone marrow specimens may establish the diagnosis by demonstrating granulomatous inflammation with organisms visible on special stains, or by yielding the bacteria on culture. In this patient with miliary tuberculosis, a granuloma lies in the center of the field, and some caseous necrosis (the pink granular material) is visible within it.

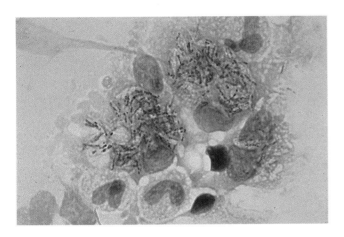

Slide 167. Mycobacteria: Special Stains of Bone Marrow Aspirate

In this patient with AIDS, fever, and pancytopenia, an acid-fast stain of a bone marrow aspirate reveals numerous beaded acid-fast (red) bacilli within the cytoplasm of macrophages. Culture of the specimen yielded *Mycobacterium avium-intracellulare.*

VIRUSES

Infectious Mononucleosis

The Epstein-Barr virus, part of the herpesvirus group, infects most humans sometime during their lives. In young children, infection with this organism is either asymptomatic or lacks distinctive clinical features, but in older children and adults a characteristic syndrome, infectious mononucleosis, develops. In tropical countries, most infections occur before age 10, and infectious mononucleosis is rare. In more affluent societies, however, a substantial percentage of adolescents and young adults are susceptible, and the disease commonly occurs between the ages of 17 and 25 years. The organism is transmitted by saliva, usually from a carrier rather than someone acutely infected. Kissing is probably the most frequent mode of infection, and the incubation period is about 3–7 weeks.

The commonest symptoms of infectious mononucleosis are anorexia, fatigue, sweats, fever, nausea, headache, sore throat, and dysphagia, in various combinations and sequences. Fever is frequent and sometimes reaches 40°C or more. Bilateral lymph node enlargement, especially affecting the cervical chain, but also commonly the axillary and inguinal nodes, is nearly universal sometime in the course of illness. The pharynx is usually inflamed, often with a patchy exudate, and erythematous palatal macules may appear. Periorbital edema may develop. Splenomegaly is detectable in about 50–75% of patients, typically in the second week of illness, and may cause left upper quadrant discomfort or early satiety. Hepatomegaly is apparent in a minority of patients.

The Epstein-Barr virus infects epithelial cells in the pharynx and B-cells. The abnormal ("atypical") lymphocytes visible on a blood smear, however, are activated T-cells that the infection has provoked. The leukocyte count is typically between 10,000 and 20,000/mm³, with 60% or more being mononuclear cells, of which at least 10% are the "atypical" lymphocytes. Mild thrombocytopenia (100,000–150,000/mm³) is common. Bone marrow examination, rarely necessary, is typically unremarkable or reveals generalized hyperplasia.

Other laboratory findings include abnormal liver tests, such as mild elevations in transaminases, alkaline phosphatase, and bilirubin. Serum LDH levels are characteristically increased. Serologic tests for specific antibodies to several antigens on the Epstein-Barr virus can establish the diagnosis of infectious mononucleosis. More commonly, the confirmatory test is the detection of the heterophil antibody, an IgM that causes agglutination of sheep and horse erythrocytes. It usually becomes positive by the second or third week of illness and disappears in 4–8 weeks. A rapid, reliable slide test is the Monospot.

Hematologic complications occur in <5% of cases. A hemolytic anemia with positive cold agglutinins (IgM) is usually mild. Severe thrombocytopenia, neutropenia, and marrow aplasia are rare. Occasionally infectious mononucleosis leads to a virus-associated hemophagocytic syndrome characterized by fever, pancytopenia, generalized lymph node enlargement, and hepatosplenomegaly. Bone marrow examination reveals hypercellular or hypocellular hematopoiesis and erythrophagocytosis by histiocytes.

Serious nonhematologic complications may also ensue, but are rare. The spleen may rupture, usually following trauma, sometimes apparently mild. Upper airway obstruction can develop from pharyngeal edema or enlargement of tonsils and other lymphatic tissue. Liver failure occasionally occurs, as may neurologic complications, including Guillain-Barré syndrome, peripheral neuropathies, aseptic meningitis, meningoencephalitis, cerebellar ataxia, cranial nerve palsies, and optic neuritis. Pericarditis and myocarditis rarely develop. For the vast majority of patients, however, infectious mononucleosis is a mild, self-limited disease that resolves within a few weeks, leaving no sequelae.

Human Immunodeficiency Virus (HIV) Infection

The clinical constellations of HIV infection are covered extensively in the infectious disease literature. Lymphocyte (particularly T-cell) numbers and functions undergo progressive impairment. These can lead to secondary infections by organisms that usually are nonpathogens, secondary malignancies, abnormal immune-mediated phenomena such as immune thrombocytopenic purpura, neutropenia and hypoproliferative anemia. Anti-HIV medications and antibiotics can also affect the blood and marrow. Marrow abnormalities in HIV infection are either nonspecific or attributable to secondary infection or an HIV-related neoplasia such as lymphoma or Kaposi's sarcoma. The nonspecific marrow findings in HIV infection include plasmacytosis, lymphocytosis (often seen as aggregates in biopsy), megaloblastosis, myelodysplasia, serous atrophy and fibrosis.

Slide 168. Infectious Mononucleosis

In infectious mononucleosis, a large number of atypical lymphocytes are usually visible. They are pleomorphic and vary in size, often being large. The nuclei are oval, kidney-shaped, or lobulated; frequently con-

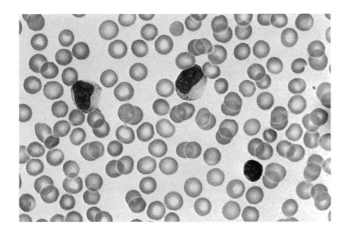

tain nucleoli; and may have diffuse, reticular, or partially condensed chromatin. The cytoplasm is often dark blue, sometimes granular or foamy, and commonly exhibits vacuolization. Where the atypical lymphocytes contact other cells, indentations may occur in the cytoplasm, with increased darkness of the edges. In most cases of infectious mononucleosis, lymphocytes constitute over half of the white cells, and at least 20% of these are atypical. When cold-antibody (IgM) hemolytic anemia occurs, the red cells may agglutinate or form rouleaux. Thrombocytopenia may also develop. Other viruses, especially cytomegalovirus, can cause a similar hematologic picture. This slide, from a patient with infectious mononucleosis, shows two large atypical lymphocytes, in which the cytoplasm is bluish-gray and the nuclei are large and oval-shaped. One normal small lymphocyte appears on the lower right, demonstrating its smaller size, rounded nucleus, and scant cytoplasm. Thrombocytopenia is also apparent.

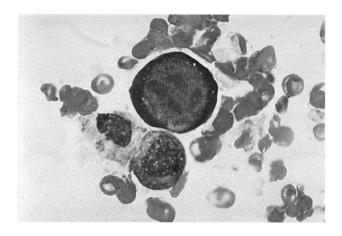

Slide 169. Parvovirus: Bone Marrow Aspirate

Parvoviruses are the smallest DNA-containing viruses that infect mammalian cells. The only known human pathogen in this group is B19, which infects most people at some time during their lives, either producing no symptoms or an illness consisting of a varying combination of fever, myalgia, arthritis, and rash, sometimes in the form of erythema infectiosum, a febrile illness with a characteristic erythema over the cheeks ("slapped cheeks") and a relative circum-oral pallor. Concurrently or a few days later, a lacy erythema often appears on the trunk and extremities. Rarely, pruritic or painful, rapidly progressive swelling and erythema develop on the hands and feet. The rash includes papules and purpura and has sharp margins at the wrists and ankles. This disorder is called "papular-purpuric gloves and socks syndrome."

The virus infects and destroys erythrocyte precursors in the bone marrow, causing red cell aplasia, which is usually short-lived and not clinically apparent unless the patient has chronic hemolysis from such disorders as sickle cell anemia or hereditary spherocytosis. Even a brief cessation of red cell production in these circumstances leads to a rapid worsening of anemia, and this organism is the most common cause of community-acquired aplastic crises. In immunodeficiency diseases, such as AIDS, the infection may become chronic, causing a sustained red cell aplasia. The characteristic bone marrow findings are a decrease in erythrocyte precursors and the presence of giant proerythroblasts, one of which is seen as the upper cell in this slide. They typically have intranuclear inclusions, four of which are present in this example. The cytoplasm is usually basophilic and contains vacuoles.

FUNGI

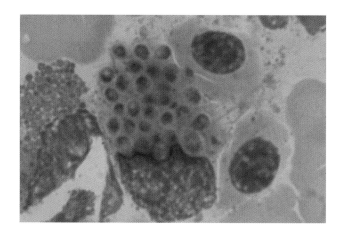

Slide 170. *Histoplasma capsulatum*: Bone Marrow Aspirate

When it causes disseminated disease, *Histoplasma capsulatum* may be visible within phagocytic cells in the bone marrow. The organisms are present as yeasts, which are round or oval, single-cell fungi that reproduce by budding. They take up Romanowsky stains, but are often better seen with periodic acid–Schiff (PAS) or Gomori's methenamine silver stains. In this aspirate, the yeasts are visible within the cytoplasm of the phagocyte in the center of the field.

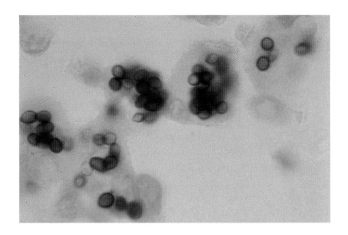

Slide 171. *Histoplasma capsulatum*: Bone Marrow Aspirate (Silver Stain)

With Gomori's methenamine silver stain, which is taken up by the fungal cell walls, the yeasts are visible as round to oval organisms, sometimes with evidence of budding. In this slide, the black, round to oval structures are the yeasts, visible within the green-staining phagocytes.

PROTOZOA

Slide 172. Malaria

All four *Plasmodium* species that cause malaria in humans—*P. falciparum, P. vivax, P. ovale,* and *P. malariae*—are visible on peripheral smears. Thick films, in

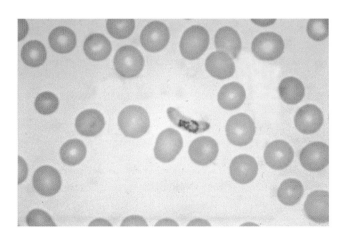

which several layers of blood are superimposed and the parasites thus concentrated, are often preferable for detecting the organisms, while thin films frequently allow better identification of the species. Several sets of blood smears from blood sampled at different times may be necessary to find the parasites. When they invade the erythrocytes, the first visible stage is a ring form, and differentiation among the species may be difficult. Later, as the organism enlarges and becomes ameboid or irregular in shape, species-specific characteristics become evident, and pigment may be detectable. Then, nuclear fission (schizogony) leads to 6–24 daughter merozoites visible within the red cells before they rupture. Some of the parasites also develop into sexual forms, gametocytes, which have distinctive features that allow species differentiation. In this slide, the banana-shaped gametocyte allows a confident diagnosis of *P. falciparum* infection to be made.

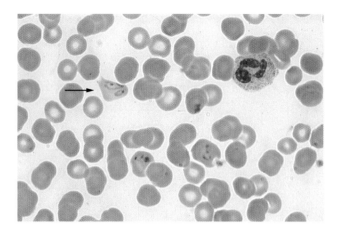

Slide 173. Malaria

This slide demonstrates several red cells containing ring forms. The nucleus of the ring form is small—a chromatin dot that stains red to purple—and the cytoplasmic ring, which stains blue, is slender. In one erythrocyte (*arrow*), two ring forms are present, which strongly suggests that this is *P. falciparum,* since the occurrence of multiple ring forms in one erythrocyte is rare in other species. Other features that can suggest *P. falciparum* are the small size and thinness of the rings, the presence of double chromatin dots, the absence of cells containing merozoites, appliqué forms (in which the ring parasites appear next to the red cell membrane), 5% or more of red cells involved, and the pathognomonic banana-shaped gametocyte, shown in the previous slide. Differentiation of this species from the others is extremely important, since *P. falciparum* malaria, a medical emergency, can be rapidly fatal without prompt, appropriate therapy. The other forms of malaria are rarely lethal.

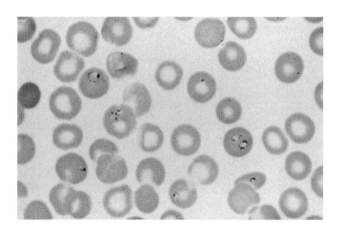

Slide 174. Babesiosis

Babesia microti, a protozoan that infects mice, is transmitted between hosts by ticks. Infected humans may be asymptomatic, but, especially in asplenic hosts, fever, myalgias, and hemolytic anemia can occur. The organisms are intraerythrocytic, ringed parasites that are 2–3 μm in diameter, have 1–2 chromatin dots, and may assume basket shapes. More than one organism can be present in a red cell; when four have their ends in contact, they form a pathognomonic Maltese cross appearance. *Babesia* organisms differ from those of malaria in that the ring forms are smaller, pigment is absent, and schizonts and gametocytes do not exist. In this slide, several of the erythrocytes contain the parasite; one in the right center contains two protozoa, while the large red cell to the left of center has four.

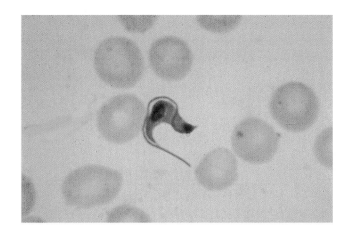

Slide 175. *Trypanosoma cruzi*

Infection with *Trypanosoma cruzi*, *T. rhodesiense*, and *T. gambiense* is often detectable by examining thin or thick blood smear preparations. American trypanosomiasis (Chagas' disease) is caused by *T. cruzi*, an organism found in Central and South America and transmitted by bites of reduviid bugs. *T. rhodesiense* and *T. gambiense*, which are morphologically identical, cause African trypanosomiasis or sleeping sickness, are found only on that continent, and are transmitted by tsetse flies. The large round purplish structure is the nucleus; the wavy thread is the flagellum, joined to the body of the organism by an undulating membrane; and the small violet dot to which the flagellum attaches at the end of the parasite is the kinetoplast. Differences in sizes of the organisms and the characteristics of their structures allow discrimination between *T. cruzi*, present in this slide, and the African species.

Slide 176. Toxoplasmosis

Toxoplasma gondii exists in three forms: tachyzoites, which indicate acute, active infection; bradyzoites in cysts, which signify latent infection; and sporozoites in oocysts, which are present only in the intestines of

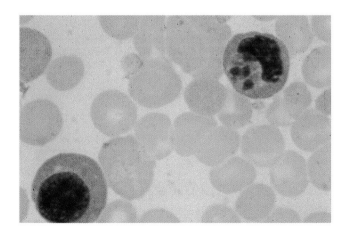

cats, the definitive hosts, or in soil contaminated by their feces. Humans become infected primarily by ingesting material contaminated with oocysts or meat containing cysts, especially pork or lamb. From these sources the tachyzoites are released in the intestines, enter the bloodstream or the lymphatics, and travel to sites where they invade tissues. Occasionally the tachyzoites are visible in the peripheral blood, but more often they or the cysts that form from them are detectable in various tissues, including the bone marrow. The tachyzoite is oval or crescent-shaped, about 3 by 7 μm in size, with a central nucleus and one end that is pointed, the other round. They may be present within any cell except non-nucleated erythrocytes. Cysts are about 10–100 μm in diameter and contain numerous bradyzoites, which are nearly identical to the tachyzoites in appearance. In this slide, two megaloblastic nucleated red cells are visible. In the one in the right upper corner, four tachyzoites lie in the cytoplasm, indenting the nucleus.

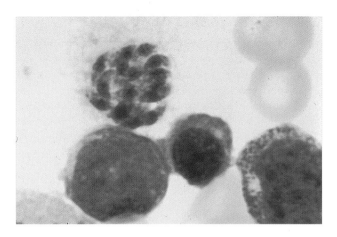

Slide 177. Toxoplasmosis: Bone Marrow Aspirate

In this bone marrow aspirate, a cyst is present with numerous bradyzoites inside. The cyst wall does not stain well with Romanowsky dyes, but it is easily visible with periodic acid–Schiff or silver stains.

FILARIA

Adult filarial parasites live in subcutaneous tissues or lymphatics and reproduce sexually to generate microfilaria, which may be visible in the bloodstream or bone marrow aspirates. Some (*Wuchereria bancrofti*, *Brugia malayi*, *Mansonella perstans*) characteristically release the microfilaria at night, some (*Loa loa*) during the day, and others (*Mansonella ozzardi*) at any time.

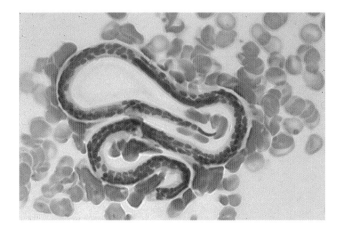

Slide 178. *Wuchereria bancrofti*: Bone Marrow Aspirate

Filariasis due to *Wuchereria bancrofti*, a mosquito-borne disease, is widespread throughout tropical countries. The microfilariae have encircling sheaths and are about 200–300 μm in length and 8 μm in diameter. The purple circles throughout the organism are called body nuclei. The size and curvature of the microfilaria, the presence or absence of a sheath, the nature of the body nuclei, and the characteristics of the tail distinguish among the various species of microfilariae. In this slide, the microfilaria lies coiled among numerous erythrocytes.

Miscellaneous Disorders

HEMATOLOGIC EFFECTS OF ALCOHOLISM

Excessive alcohol intake may produce hematologic abnormalities indirectly because of associated malnutrition (e.g., folic acid deficiency), liver disease (e.g., spur-cell anemia), or gastrointestinal hemorrhage (i.e., anemia from acute bleeding or from iron deficiency caused by chronic blood loss). Alcohol, however, has direct hematologic effects as well, including several bone marrow findings. Vacuolization of the hematopoietic precursors, especially in the cytoplasm of proerythroblasts, occurs frequently with high intake, appearing within 1 week of the onset of heavy drinking and vanishing a few days after abstinence. Vacuoles can form in the nuclei of proerythroblasts and the cytoplasm of promyelocytes. Reversible hypocellularity of the bone marrow or megaloblastic changes in the absence of other causes occasionally occur, and the marrow may also show an unexplained increase in plasma cells. Ringed sideroblasts may form, and these commonly disappear days to weeks following sobriety. The mechanism may involve impaired pyridoxine or iron metabolism or a direct effect of alcohol on heme biosynthesis. Occasionally a macrocytic or microcytic anemia develops in association with the sideroblasts.

About 60% of alcoholics have a macrocytosis attributable to alcohol alone, with the MCV usually 100–110 fl. The characteristic findings of macro-ovalocytes and hypersegmented neutrophils seen in folate or vitamin B_{12} deficiency are absent, as is anemia, unless another disorder coexists. The macrocytosis persists until 2–4 months after abstinence. Target cells and stomatocytes may also be visible on blood smears. Excessive alcohol intake sometimes causes thrombocytopenia, which usually subsides within a few days of sobriety, but may "overcorrect" to cause a transient thrombocytosis in 1–3 weeks. The number of megakaryocytes in the bone marrow may be normal or reduced.

Severe neutropenia may occur in alcoholics, typically associated with a severe bacterial infection. In these patients the bone marrow demonstrates hypocellularity with decreased mature granulocytes. Other reasons for neutropenia include folate deficiency and hypersplenism. Neutropenia without an apparent cause other than alcoholism may also occur; in these patients the marrow is usually normal except for vacuoles in the erythroid and granulocyte precursors. Excessive alcohol intake can also cause lymphocytopenia.

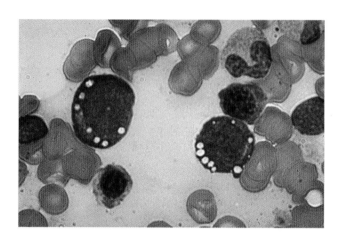

Slide 179. Effects of Alcoholism: Bone Marrow Aspirate

The two proerythroblasts in this slide, from a patient with alcoholism, show numerous cytoplasmic vacuoles.

METASTATIC CANCER

Many malignancies metastasize to the bone marrow. Among adults, the most common sites of origin are carcinomas of the lung, breast, and prostate. A single trephine bone marrow biopsy recovers malignant cells in about one-third to one-half of cases in which osseous metastases are present. Obtaining bilateral iliac crest specimens increases the yield. About one-half to three-quarters of patients with positive biopsies have a positive bone marrow aspirate. This lower diagnostic rate arises partly from the frequent presence of fibrosis (desmoplastic response) around malignant cells, which makes them difficult to aspirate. In less than half of the cases of bone marrow metastases, leukoerythroblastosis occurs on the peripheral blood smear; its presence correlates more with the amount of marrow fibrosis than with the extent of malignancy. In many patients with bone marrow metastases, the peripheral blood smear is completely normal.

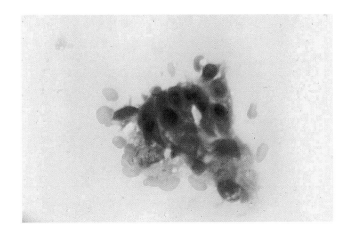

Slide 180. Metastatic Lung Cancer: Bone Marrow Aspirate

On bone marrow aspirates, metastatic cells often clump. Usually larger than hematopoietic cells, except megakaryocytes, they are commonly pleomorphic. The nuclear-cytoplasmic ratio is frequently high, mitoses may be plentiful, nucleoli are frequently present, and the nuclei are often hyperchromic, with a fine chromatin. The precise site of origin of the primary tumor is usually impossible to determine confidently, but certain characteristics of the cell type are suggestive, such as clear cells indicating a probable renal source and the presence of melanin pigment indicating a metastatic melanoma. In response to the metastases, osteoblasts and osteoclasts may be present. Sometimes the tumor provokes nonspecific reactions that can include increased granulocytes, megakaryocytes, plasma cells, or eosinophils. In this slide, a poorly preserved cluster of malignant cells arising from a lung primary lies in the center of the field. Such degenerative features are common in aspirate smears of metastatic malignancy. The neoplastic cells in this slide are large, have very little cytoplasm, and possess pleomorphic nuclei.

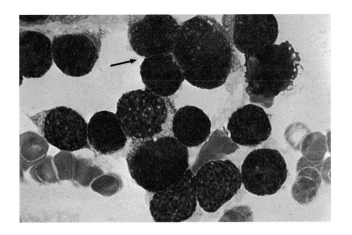

Slide 181. Metastatic Small-Cell Cancer of the Lung: Bone Marrow Aspirate

The malignant cells in this slide have large nuclei with dispersed chromatin, little cytoplasm, and variable sizes. There are several degenerating cells, a feature common in aspirates of metastatic malignancy. The nuclear borders may be smudged, and loss of the cytoplasm can cause the cells to resemble blasts. The *arrow* points to "nuclear molding," a feature seen in small-cell carcinoma.

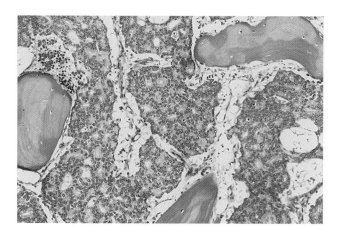

Slide 182. Metastatic Breast Carcinoma: Bone Marrow Biopsy

Metastases are diffuse or focal on bone marrow biopsy, and, especially when the infiltrate is large, central necrosis can occur. Osteolytic tumors lead to loss of bony trabeculae. With osteoblastic metastases, such as from prostate and breast cancer, new bone formation and numerous osteoblasts may be prominent. Adenocarcinomas originating from any site can form glands and mucin. In this slide, from a patient with metastatic breast carcinoma, large sheets of malignant cells cluster in glandlike aggregates.

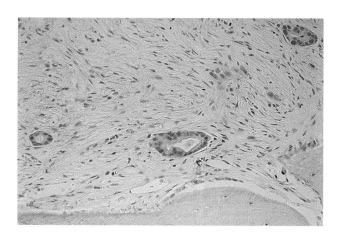

Slide 183. Metastatic Adenocarcinoma with Fibrosis: Bone Marrow Biopsy

Some malignancies provoke substantial fibrosis when they involve bone marrow. This "desmoplastic" response is most common with tumors originating from the breast, lung, stomach, and prostate. In this slide, several foci of malignant cells form glandlike structures within a large area of fibrous tissue above the bony trabecula. (The fibrosis should be compared with that in slide 87.) Because of the fibrosis, the peripheral smear may exhibit the findings of a "myelophthisic" disorder, as occurs when abnormal tissue infiltrates normal marrow. These changes include leukoerythroblastosis (see slide 29), polychromatophilia, and teardrop cells.

STORAGE DISEASES

Gaucher's Disease

Gaucher's disease is an autosomal recessive disorder found predominantly but not exclusively in people of Ashkenazi Jewish descent. The homozygous state causes a deficiency in a lysosomal enzyme, glucocerebrosidase, needed to degrade glucocerebroside, which is released from dying cells such as neutrophils. Macrophages ingest the insoluble glucocerebroside, and the accumulation of macrophages in liver, spleen, bone marrow, and occasionally other organs leads to the clinical features. Of the three kinds of Gaucher's disease, type 1, the "adult" form, is the most common; its manifestations can become apparent in childhood or later in life. The spleen is often massive and may cause abdominal discomfort and pancytopenia. Chronic fatigue is frequent. Bone pain, sometimes severe and often the most prominent symptom, can arise from infarction or pathologic fractures, primarily from osteolytic lesions in the long bones but also in the ribs, pelvis, and vertebrae. A characteristic early change is an osteolytic lesion in the distal femur that resembles an Erlenmeyer flask. Aseptic necrosis of the femoral heads can occur. Hepatic enlargement, sometimes causing abdominal discomfort, is also common, and liver fibrosis can lead to portal hypertension.

A normochromic, normocytic anemia is frequently seen, but usually the hematocrit exceeds 25. Leukopenia is typically mild, but thrombocytopenia can be severe, leading to bleeding complications. With hepatic involvement, liver enzyme levels rise and the prothrombin time lengthens. Serum acid phosphatase is usually increased. Gaucher cells, characteristically present in the bone marrow, liver, and spleen, have small eccentric nuclei surrounded by a crinkled or striated cytoplasm containing the glucocerebroside. The definitive way to establish the presence of Gaucher's disease is to measure glucocerebrosidase activity in the patient's leukocytes or fibroblasts or to detect the known mutations in the patient's DNA.

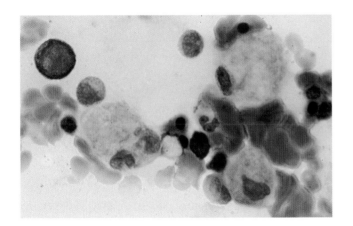

Slide 184. Gaucher's Disease: Bone Marrow Aspirate

Many patients with Gaucher's disease have no hematologic abnormalities. When abnormalities do occur, they result from hypersplenism, which can cause pancytopenia or an isolated reduction in any cell line. Since the definitive diagnosis rests on the studies mentioned above, bone marrow samples are unnecessary, but they usually reveal the characteristic Gaucher cell, which has a small, eccentric nucleus and an abundant pale-blue cytoplasm with a crinkled or striated appearance. Cells indistinguishable on light microscopy from Gaucher cells sometimes occur in other disorders, such as lymphomas, chronic granulocytic leukemia, and multiple myeloma, because increased cell turnover exceeds the normal catabolic capacity of glucocerebrosidase. Usually the underlying diagnosis is evident from the abundance of tumor cells in the bone marrow sample. In this slide, three typical Gaucher cells are present.

SARCOIDOSIS

In sarcoidosis, a disease of unknown cause, the involved organs contain noncaseating granulomas, sometimes accompanied by fibrosis. This disorder can occur in virtually any part of the body, but the vast majority of patients have disease in the thoracic cavity, affecting the lung parenchyma and lymph nodes in the mediastinum and hila, usually bilaterally. Other areas commonly involved include the eyes and skin. The usual age at onset is between 20 and 40, with rates about 10 times higher among blacks than whites in the United States. The disease is generally more common in females than males, but its frequency varies considerably in countries throughout the world. Sarcoidosis is more common in northern than southern Europe and is relatively unusual in Asia and South America, where it is more prevalent in colder than warmer climates. The duration and prognosis relate to the onset and extent of disease: patients with the abrupt onset of erythema nodosum or with asymptomatic bilateral hilar lymph node enlargement tend to have a short, self-limited course, while those with insidious onset and extensive extrapulmonary involvement often have progressive fibrosis of the lungs and other organs.

Hematologic abnormalities are common in sarcoidosis. Anemia occurs in about 5–30% of cases; its cause may be hypersplenism, present in approximately 15% of patients; anemia of chronic disease; granulomas in the bone marrow, causing replacement or suppression of hematopoietic cells; immune-related hemolysis (rarely); or apparently unrelated conditions, such as iron deficiency. The red cells are usually normochromic and normocytic, and the anemia typically resolves with systemic corticosteroid therapy. Neutropenia (defined as <3,000 neutrophils/mm^3) occurs in about 30–40% of patients, but is usually mild. The most likely cause is the presence of bone marrow granulomas. Lymphopenia (<1,500 lymphocytes/mm^3) develops in 30–50% of cases, commonly with reduced T-lymphocyte numbers and CD4/CD8 ratios, and may originate as lymphocytes migrate out of the circulation into areas of inflammation. Eosinophilia (>250 eosinophils/mm^3) develops in 5–35% of patients through unknown mechanisms. Monocytosis (>800 monocytes/mm^3) occurs in about 10% of cases. Thrombocytopenia, an uncommon finding, can arise from hypersplenism or immunologic destruction.

The bone marrow biopsy discloses granulomas in about one-half of patients with anemia. Usually disease is clinically evident in many other sites, especially in the thoracic cavity, but chest films are sometimes normal. Typically the granulomas are numerous and well-formed but occupy only a small amount of the bone marrow specimen. Langhans' giant cells may be apparent, but necrosis is very rare and should strongly suggest another diagnosis.

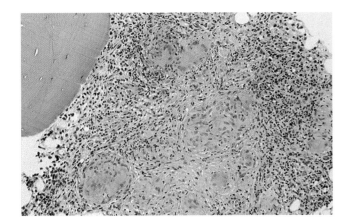

Slide 185. Sarcoidosis: Bone Marrow Biopsy

This slide discloses several noncaseating granulomas with giant cells admixed with reactive inflammatory cells, including a prominent population of small lymphocytes.

FINDINGS FOLLOWING SPLENECTOMY

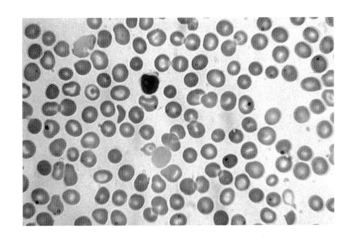

Slide 186. Splenectomy: Peripheral Smear

In the first week after splenectomy, neutrophilia is common, but it generally abates. Mild to moderate leukocytosis may persist, usually because of increased lymphocytes and monocytes rather than neutrophils. Beginning about one week after splenectomy, many patients have marked thrombocytosis, sometimes up to $2,000 \times 10^9$/L (2 million/mm^3), but the platelet count then typically falls to levels of about $500–1,000 \times 10^9$/L, which may persist for years. Platelets may also be larger than normal. Changes in the erythrocytes are universal. Howell-Jolly bodies are present in varying numbers in all patients, and Pappenheimer bodies are also frequent. The red cell surface area increases, commonly leading to target cells. Abnormal cells that the spleen ordinarily removes, such as acanthocytes, spherocytes, and bizarre-shaped erythrocytes, are often present. Similarly, polychromatophilic cells are numerous; the spleen ordinarily removes many of these from the circulation until they mature. In this slide, several Howell-Jolly bodies are present, along with target cells, spherocytes, and polychromatophilic erythrocytes. This patient also had hypothyroidism, which may explain the macrocytosis.

SYSTEMIC MAST CELL DISEASE

In this disorder, excessive mast cells infiltrate various organs, most frequently the skin, bone marrow, liver, lymph nodes, spleen, and gastrointestinal tract. About 65% of cases occur in childhood, and in most of these patients the disease resolves or markedly improves during adolescence. When the disease begins in adults, the average age at onset is about 60, and both sexes are equally affected. A classification of systemic mastocytosis defines four groups: indolent disease, by far the most common form; mastocytosis associated with a hematologic disorder; aggressive lymph node involvement with blood eosinophilia; and mast cell leukemia. Skin lesions in the form of urticaria pigmentosa may be present in any of the four forms. Characteristic are numerous reddish-brown, macular or slightly raised lesions several millimeters in diameter, primarily on the trunk and proximal extremities. They may cause pruritus and dermographism. A pathognomonic feature is Darier's sign, the development of a wheal on rubbing or scratching the lesion.

In indolent disease, the other findings related to infiltration of organs by mast cells are skeletal disease, hepatosplenomegaly, lymph node enlargement, malabsorption from small intestinal invasion, and hematologic abnormalities resulting from bone marrow involvement. Skeletal disease includes diffuse osteopenia or focal sclerotic or lytic lesions; these bony abnormalities may be asymptomatic or may cause pain or fractures. Many patients have some laboratory evidence of fat malabsorption, but it is usually insufficiently severe to produce significant clinical findings. Excessive mast cells in the bone marrow, present in about 90% of patients, result in anemia in about 30–50%, thrombocytopenia in 15–20%, leukopenia in 15–20%, leukocytosis in 20–30%, and eosinophilia in up to 40%.

Other manifestations of indolent disease originate from the systemic effects of mast cell mediators, either stored within cytoplasmic granules or produced at the time of mast cell stimulation. These include histamine; eicosanoids, such as prostaglandin 2; and cytokines, including tumor necrosis factor and various interleukins. Their hemodynamic effects may cause syncope or flushing, and their gastrointestinal effects include diarrhea and increased gastric acidity, which sometimes leads to peptic ulcers of the stomach and duodenum. Patients may have constitutional complaints such as fever, malaise, and weight loss, while neurologic effects include headaches and confusion. Many of the symptoms caused by mast cell mediators appear or worsen with exercise, heat, alcohol, narcotics, salicylates, and anticholinergic agents.

In the second type of mast cell disease, patients have a concurrent hematologic condition, most commonly a myelodysplastic or myeloproliferative disease. Other associated malignancies have included Hodgkin's disease or non-Hodgkin's lymphoma and various leukemias, some secondary to a previously underlying hematologic disease. Fever, weight loss, gastrointestinal complaints, pruritus, dermographism, and flushing are more common in this type than in the indolent form. The prognosis for the patient depends primarily on the associated disease, however, rather than on the mastocytosis itself.

The third type of systemic mast cell disease is an aggressive disorder, with lymph node enlargement affecting both peripheral and intra-abdominal sites, hepatosplenomegaly, and peripheral eosinophilia, leading to a markedly shortened survival. Ascites may be present.

The fourth type, mast cell leukemia, is defined by the presence of at least 10% mast cells, many hypogranular or multinucleated, among the circulating nucleated cell population. Skin lesions are usually absent, and the patients typically have fever, weight loss, weakness, hepatosplenomegaly, and gastrointestinal symptoms of abdominal pain, vomiting, and diarrhea.

Evaluation of a patient for the presence of systemic mast cell disease should involve a careful skin examination and biopsies of suspicious lesions; bone marrow aspiration and biopsy; serum tryptase level determinations (often increased); and 24-hour urine collections for mediators such as histamine. Biopsies of clinically involved tissues such as lymph nodes or intestinal mucosa may demonstrate increased populations of mast cells, whose reliable detection requires special stains, such as Giemsa and toluidine blue, or monoclonal antibodies to tryptase or chymase.

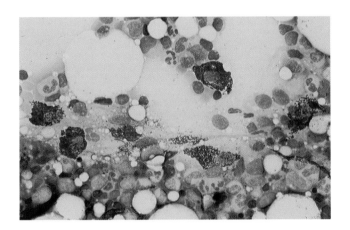

Slide 187. Systemic Mast Cell Disease: Bone Marrow Aspirate, Toluidine Blue Stain

In systemic mast cell disease the peripheral blood is often normal, but increased numbers of some cells may occur, such as eosinophils, basophils, monocytes, neutrophils, and platelets. Mast cells are visible in the peripheral blood in patients with mast cell leukemia. On the aspirate, mast cells are often increased and may be cytologically normal, exhibiting the characteristic purplish granules in the cytoplasm and a central nucleus. Sometimes, however, they are atypical in having a lobulated nucleus or decreased granules. Mast cells stain, as in this slide, with a metachromatic preparation, toluidine blue, and appear as heavily granulated cells, commonly in the bone marrow stroma.

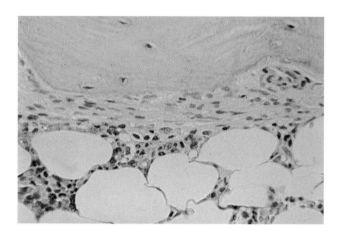

Slide 188. Systemic Mast Cell Disease: Bone Marrow Biopsy

On biopsy, the mast cells commonly provoke extensive fibrosis and are most frequent around blood vessels, adjacent to bony trabeculae, or in small nodules. Occasionally, mast cells diffusely replace the bone marrow. They are usually spindle- or oval-shaped cells with clear cytoplasm. Eosinophils, lymphocytes, and plasma cells may accompany the mast cells. In other portions of the marrow, increases in granulocytes, eosinophils, and megakaryocytes are common. In this slide, spindle-shaped mast cells lie below the bony trabecula.

Index

Note: Page numbers followed by the letter f refer to figures and those followed by t refer to tables.